THE
Sugarless Cookbook

Volume 2

COOKING WITH THE NATURAL SWEETNESS OF FRUIT

by Nellie G. Hum

Front Cover: Black Forest Cake, page 80

The Sugarless Cookbook, Volume 2
by Nellie G. Hum

Second Printing - August 1992

Copyright © 1985 by
Nellie G. Hum

Hum Publishing
395 Second Avenue
Ottawa, Ontario
Canada K1S 2J3

All rights reserved. Except for reviews, no part of this book may be reproduced without permission from the publisher.

Canadian Cataloguing in Publication Data

Hum, Nellie G.

The sugarless cookbook

Contents: v.2. Cooking with the natural sweetness of fruit.
ISBN 0-919845-97-5 (vol. 2)

1. Sugar-free diet — Recipes. 2. Cookery (Fruit).
I. Title.
RM237.85.H85 1987   641.5/63   C87-098041-6

Photography by
Patricia Holdsworth
Patricia Holdsworth Photography
Regina, Saskatchewan

Designed, Printed and Produced in Canada by
Centax Books, A Division of M•C•Graphics Inc.
Publishing Director, Photo Designer and Food Stylist: Margo Embury
1048 Fleury Street
Regina, Saskatchewan, Canada   S4N 4W8
(306)359-3737 FAX (306) 525-3955

TABLE OF CONTENTS

Introduction	4
Muffins and Pancakes	5
Yeast Breads, Buns and Cakes	10
Salad and Fruit Dressings	21
Vegetables	25
Main Dishes	32
Sauces, Relishes and Pickles	46
Jams and Sweet Sauces	57
Pastry and Pies	62
Puddings and Cheesecakes	71
Cakes	80
Cookies, Bars and Squares	94
Treats	102
Index	107

Recipes have been tested in U.S. standard measurements. Common metric measurements are given as a convenience for those who are more familiar with metric. Recipes have not been tested in metric.

INTRODUCTION

Ever since the inception of the first *Sugarless Cookbook*, I have been overwhelmed with the amount of interest in cooking without sugar. Your many letters and telephone calls have informed me of your wish for more recipes using the natural sweetness of fruit juices and fruits.

Encouraged by your enthusiasm, I was prompted to write *The Sugarless Cookbook Volume 2*. As in Volume 1 only fruits and fruit juices, instead of sugar, honey, molasses, corn syrup, cyclamates or aspartames, are used to sweeten all recipes. Wherever possible, vegetable oil is suggested instead of solid fats and the use of salt is minimized.

You will find an array of chiffon cakes, yeast recipes, pickles, jams and ketchup. With the popularity of chocolate, there is Black Forest Cake, Chocolate-Dipped Fruit and more. For those who prefer carob, simply substitute the same amount of carob for chocolate and vice versa. The Rhubarb Pie and all other pies are made with a single crust. The suggested toppings are decorative and tasty, without the extra calories of a double-crust pie. In addition to desserts, a range of main dishes, usually requiring sugar, is featured, using fruit juices instead.

I appreciate all your cheerful and encouraging messages. It is my hope that I have answered some of your requests, if not all.

CANNED FRUIT AND FRUIT JUICES:

Read labels for sugar content when buying canned goods. **Unsweetened** fruit packed in its own juice, or in any other juice, should be used whenever canned fruit is required in these recipes.

Unsweetened fruit juices and **unsweetened** concentrated fruit juices have been used in recipes throughout this book. If unsweetened concentrated **pineapple** juice is unavailable, substitute unsweetened concentrated **apple** juice.

Muffins and Pancakes

PUMPKIN MUFFINS

Preheat oven to 375°F (190°C). Mix together in a mixing bowl:

2 cups	(	500 mL)	all-purpose OR whole-wheat flour
3 tsp.	(	15 mL)	baking powder
½ tsp.	(	2 mL)	baking soda
1 tsp.	(	5 mL)	cinnamon
½ tsp.	(	2 mL)	nutmeg
¼ tsp.	(	1 mL)	ginger
⅛ tsp.	(	0.5 mL)	cloves

Add and mix well:

| ½ cup | (| 125 mL) | chopped walnuts |
| ½ cup | (| 125 mL) | raisins |

Cream until soft:

| 6 tbsp. | (| 90 mL) | butter OR margarine |

Beat in:

| 1 | (| 1) | large egg |

Add and beat until blended:

| 1 cup | (| 250 mL) | mashed, cooked OR canned pumpkin |
| ⅓ cup | (| 75 mL) | unsweetened concentrated apple juice, room temperature |

Add egg mixture to dry ingredients. Stir just enough to moisten flour. Fill greased muffin cups ⅔ full. Bake until golden, about 25 minutes. Makes 12 muffins.

BANANA-NUT BRAN MUFFINS

Preheat oven to 375°F (190°C). Combine in a mixing bowl:
- 1 cup (250 mL) all-purpose OR whole-wheat flour
- 2 tsp. (10 mL) baking powder
- ¾ tsp. (4 mL) baking soda

Add and mix well:
- 1½ cups (375 mL) natural bran
- ½ cup (125 mL) chopped walnuts

Beat until blended:
- 1 (1) large egg, beaten
- 2 tbsp. (30 mL) melted butter, margarine OR oil
- 1 cup (250 mL) mashed ripe bananas
- 6 tbsp. (90 mL) unsweetened concentrated apple juice, room temperature

Add liquid mixture to dry ingredients. Stir just enough to moisten flour. Fill greased muffin cups ⅔ full. Bake until golden brown, about 25 minutes. Makes 12 muffins.

See photograph on page 16A.

OATMEAL MUFFINS

Preheat oven to 400°F (200°C). Mix together; set aside until cool:
- ¾ cup (175 mL) milk, hot
- 2 tsp. (10 mL) lemon juice
- 4 tbsp. (60 mL) unsweetened concentrated fruit juice, any flavour, defrosted
- 1 cup (250 mL) quick-cooking rolled oats

Combine in a mixing bowl:
- 1¼ cups (300 mL) whole-wheat OR all-purpose flour
- 1 tsp. (5 mL) baking powder
- 1 tsp. (5 mL) baking soda
- 1 tsp. (5 mL) cinnamon

Mix in:
- ⅓ cup (75 mL) chopped walnuts OR raisins

OATMEAL MUFFINS (continued)

Beat until blended:

    1 (1)   egg, beaten
2 tbsp. (30 mL)   melted butter, margarine OR oil

Stir cooled mixture into egg mixture. Add to dry ingredients, stirring just enough to moisten flour. Fill greased muffin cups ⅔ full. Bake until done, 20-25 minutes. Makes 12 muffins.

See photograph on page 16A.

RICE-RAISIN MUFFINS

Preheat oven to 400°F (200°C). Mix together in a mixing bowl:

1½ cups (375 mL) whole-wheat OR all-purpose flour
3 tsp. (15 mL) baking powder
½ tsp. (2 mL) baking soda
1 tsp. (5 mL) cinnamon
½ cup (125 mL) raisins

Combine:

    1 (1)   egg, beaten
2 tbsp. (30 mL) melted butter, margarine OR oil
1 cup (250 mL) milk

Combine and add:

1 cup (250 mL) cooked rice
4 tbsp. (60 mL) unsweetened concentrated apple juice, room temperature.

Stir egg mixture lightly into flour mixture, just to moisten. Fill greased muffin cups ⅔ full. Bake until browned, 20-25 minutes. Serve hot. Makes 12 muffins.

See photograph on page 16A.

RICE-BACON MUFFINS

From above recipe, omit cinnamon and raisins. Into juice stir:

    6 (6)   slices crisp-cooked bacon, crumbled

RICE PANCAKES

Sift together:
- ¾ cup (175 mL) whole-wheat OR all-purpose flour
- 1 tsp. (5 mL) baking powder
- ¼ tsp. (1 mL) baking soda

Combine:
- ¾ cup (175 mL) milk
- 1 cup (250 mL) cooked rice

Beat until blended:
- 1 (1) egg, beaten
- 1 tbsp. (15 mL) melted butter, margarine OR oil
- 4 tbsp. (60 mL) unsweetened concentrated apple juice, room temperature

Beat rice mixture into egg mixture. Add flour mixture; stir just until blended. For each pancake, pour 2 tbsp. (30 mL) of batter onto a hot lightly oiled griddle. When covered with bubbles, turn and brown other side. Serve hot with butter or margarine and any sweet sauce, pages 57-61. Makes twelve 3¼" (8 cm) pancakes.

MEXICAN CRÊPES

Beat until blended:
- 2 (2) eggs, beaten
- 4 tbsp. (60 mL) cornmeal
- 3 tbsp. (45 mL) flour (unbleached, whole-wheat OR all-purpose)
- ¾ cup (175 mL) milk
- ¼ cup (60 mL) unsweetened apple juice

Let stand 15 minutes. Stir and measure 2 tbsp. (30 mL) batter into a hot oiled 6" (15 cm) frying pan. Rotate pan quickly to spread batter over the bottom. Brown both sides. Serve with butter or margarine and syrup or any sweet sauce, pages 57-61. Crêpes may also be used as a wrap for meat or savoury fillings. Makes 10 crêpes.

CHOCOLATE DESSERT PANCAKES

Sift together:
- 1 cup (250 mL) all-purpose flour
- 5 tbsp. (75 mL) cocoa
- 1½ tsp. (7 mL) baking powder
- ½ tsp. (2 mL) baking soda

Beat together:
- 1 (1) egg, beaten
- 1 tbsp. (15 mL) vegetable oil
- ¾ cup (175 mL) milk

Add to egg mixture:
- ¾ cup (175 mL) unsweetened concentrated fruit juice, any flavour, defrosted

Stir flour mixture into egg mixture until smooth. Add:
- ¼ cup (60 mL) coarsely chopped nuts

Make small pancakes by pouring 1 tbsp. (15 mL) of batter onto a hot lightly oiled griddle for each pancake. Cook until the tops are covered with bubbles; turn and cook other side. Allow 2 pancakes per serving; top each with:

Low-Calorie Chocolate Topping, recipe follows, OR Chocolate Whipped Cream, page 85

Make twenty-six 2¾"(7 cm) pancakes.

LOW-CALORIE CHOCOLATE TOPPING

Combine:
- 2 tbsp. (30 mL) unsweetened concentrated apple juice, defrosted
- ½ tsp. (2 mL) vanilla
- 1¼ tsp. (6 mL) gelatine

Mix together:
- 1 tsp. (5 mL) cocoa
- 2 tsp. (10 mL) hot water

Add cocoa mixture to gelatine mixture. Warm over low heat until gelatine dissolves completely. Gradually stir in:
- ½ cup (125 mL) evaporated milk, 2% m.f.

Chill until thickened but not set. Beat until light and fluffy. Makes 1 cup (250 mL).

Yeast Breads, Buns and Cakes

LEMON-RAISIN BUNDT CAKE

With a pastry brush, brush oil inside a 3-quart (3 L) nonstick bundt pan.

Cream until soft and creamy:
- ¾ cup (175 mL) **butter OR margarine**
- **grated rind of 2 small lemons OR 1 large lemon**
- ¼ tsp. (1 mL) **salt**

Warm over low heat to 105-115°F (40-45°C):
- 4 tbsp. (60 mL) **unsweetened apple juice**

Sprinkle with:
- 1 tbsp. (15 mL) **active dry yeast (1 pkg.)**

Let stand until surface is foamy, 10 minutes; stir with a fork to moisten any dry particles.

With an electric beater, beat into the creamed mixture, 1 at a time:
- 2 (2) **egg yolks**
- 2 (2) **whole eggs**

Beat in the yeast mixture. Add and beat until blended:
- 1½ cups (375mL) **all-purpose flour**

Warm over low heat to 105-115°F (40-45°C):
- ¾ cup (175 mL) **unsweetened concentrated apple juice, defrosted**

To the yeast mixture add the warm juice and:
- 1½ cups (375 mL) **all-purpose flour**

LEMON-RAISIN BUNDT CAKE (continued)

Beat on low speed until thoroughly blended. Mix in:
    1 cup   (**250 mL**)   **raisins**

Spread dough in bundt pan; smooth top with spatula. Cover with plastic wrap. Let rise in a warm, 80-85°F (27-30°C), place until doubled; remove plastic wrap before dough touches it. Bake in middle of oven at 400°F (200°C) for 5 minutes. Lower to 350°F (180°C) and bake 25 minutes. Cool 10 minutes. Remove cake by placing wire rack over bundt pan, turn to unmould. Cool 1½ hours. Serves 12.

APPLE-CHEDDAR COFFEE CAKE

Combine:
    1 tbsp.   (**15 mL**)   **unsweetened concentrated apple juice, defrosted**
    1 tbsp.   (**15 mL**)   **boiling water**

Cool to 105-115°F (40-45°C).

Sprinkle with:
    1½ tsp.   (**7 mL**)   **active dry yeast (½ pkg.)**

Let stand until surface is foamy, 10 minutes; stir with fork to moisten any dry particles.

Cream until soft and creamy:
    4 tbsp.   (**60 mL**)   **butter OR margarine**
    ¼ tsp.   (**1 mL**)   **salt**

With an electric beater, beat into the butter mixture the yeast mixture and:
    1   (**1**)   **egg**

Add:
    ⅔ cup   (**150 mL**)   **all-purpose flour**
    ½ cup   (**125 mL**)   **unsweetened concentrated apple juice, warmed to 105-115°F (40-45°C)**

APPLE COFFEE CAKE (continued)

Beat until smooth. Add:
- 1 cup (250 mL) all-purpose flour

Beat on low speed until well-blended. Cover with a damp cloth. Let rise in a warm, 80-85°F (27-30°C), place until doubled in size, about 1¼ hours. Stir down. Spread half the batter in an oiled 9" (23 cm) round cake pan. Add a layer of:
- ½ cup (125 mL) grated old Cheddar cheese (2 oz./57 g)

Add the remaining batter, then another layer of:
- ½ cup (125 mL) grated old Cheddar cheese (2 oz./57 g)

Top with a layer, arranged in a circular pattern:
- 1½ (1½) medium apples, peeled, cored and thinly sliced*

Combine:
- 2 tbsp. (30 mL) fine cracker crumbs
- 1 tsp. (5 mL) soft butter OR margarine
- 1 tsp. (5 mL) cinnamon

Sprinkle this mixture over apples. Let rise in a warm, 80-85°F (27-30°C), place until doubled, about 1 hour. Bake in the middle of the oven at 375°F (190°C) until nicely browned, about 35 minutes.

* Slice apples into quarters; cut each quarter into 4 wedges; dip each wedge into:
- 4 tsp. (20 mL) unsweetened concentrated apple juice, defrosted

Serves 8.

FOR JUICIER CITRUS FRUIT

Soak citrus fruit (oranges, lemons, grapefruits, or limes) in hot water for 10-15 minutes. This will increase the juice at least half as much more. You can also microwave citrus fruit for 30-45 seconds on 100% power to increase juice yield.

POPPY SEED RING

In a mixing bowl, combine:
- **2 tbsp.   (30 mL)   unsweetened concentrated apple juice, defrosted**
- **2 tbsp.   (30 mL)   boiling water**

Cool to 105-115°F (40-45°F).

Sprinkle with:
- **1 tbsp.   (15 mL)   active dry yeast (1 pkg.)**

Let stand until surface is foamy, 10 minutes; stir with a fork to moisten any dry particles.

In a small saucepan, combine:
- **½ cup   (125 mL)   unsweetened concentrated apple juice, defrosted**
- **4 tbsp.   (60 mL)   butter OR margarine**
- **2 tsp.   (10 mL)   grated lemon rind**
- **¼ tsp.   (1 mL)   salt**
- **¼ cup   (60 mL)   water**

Heat until butter OR margarine melts. Cool to 105-115°F (40-45°C).

Add the juice mixture to the yeast liquid, then add:
- **1   (1)   egg, well beaten**
- **1½ cups   (375 mL)   all-purpose flour**

Beat until smooth. Add and mix by hand:
- **1½ cups   (375 mL)   all-purpose flour**

When dough comes away from bowl, turn it out onto a lightly floured board. Knead until smooth and elastic, 10 minutes. Place dough in a greased mixing bowl; turn the dough over to grease the entire surface. Cover the bowl with a damp cloth. Let rise in a warm, 80-85°F (27-30°C), place until doubled, approximately 1½-2 hours. Punch down with your fist; pull the edges to the centre; turn dough out onto a lightly floured board. Cover; let rest 10 minutes. Roll dough into a rectangle, 19½" x 10" (49 x 25 cm). Spread Poppy Seed Filling, recipe follows, within ½"(1.3 cm) of the edges. Roll up dough, jelly-roll fashion, from the longest edge. Brush edge with:
- **1   (1)   egg yolk, beaten**

Press well to seal. Place roll in a 3-quart (3 L) nonstick bundt or tube pan. Brush ends with egg yolk, press firmly to join. Cover and let rise again until doubled, about 1 hour.

POPPY SEED RING (continued)

Beat with a fork, the remainder of egg yolk and:
    1 tsp.   (5 mL)   water

Brush roll with the egg wash. Sprinkle with:
                poppy seeds or sesame seeds

Bake in the middle of the oven at 400°F (200°C) for 10 minutes; reduce heat to 375°F (190°C) and bake until nicely browned, 45 minutes. Serves 8-10.

POPPY SEED FILLING

Spread on a cookie sheet:
    1 cup   (250 mL)   poppy seeds

Roast at 300°F (150°C) for 10 to 15 minutes, stirring twice for even browning. Then grind with a hand mill or pulverize in a blender or with a mortar and pestle. In a small saucepan, combine the poppy seeds and:
    1 cup   (250 mL)   raisins
    ¾ cup   (175 mL)   unsweetened concentrated apple juice, defrosted
    1 tbsp.   (15 mL)   butter OR margarine

Simmer and stir until thick and most of liquid has evaporated. Transfer the mixture into a bowl. Cool to room temperature. Mix in:
    1 tsp.   (5 mL)   almond extract

Beat until well-blended:
    1   (1)   egg

With a rubber spatula fold egg into poppy seed mixture. Cover with plastic wrap and refrigerate. Remove from refrigerator ½ hour before required.

Use in Poppy Seed Ring page 13.

HOT CROSS BUNS

Scald:
    ½ cup   (125 mL)   milk

Stir in:
    4 tbsp.   (60 mL)   butter OR margarine
    ¼ tsp.   (1 mL)   salt

Cool to 105-115°F (40-45°C). In a mixing bowl, combine:
    2 tbsp.   (30 mL)   unsweetened concentrated apple juice, defrosted
    2 tbsp.   (30 mL)   boiling water

Cool to 105-115°F (40-45°C). Sprinkle with:
    1 tbsp.   (15 mL)   active dry yeast (1 pkg.)

Let stand until surface is foamy, about 10 minutes; stir with fork to moisten any dry particles. To yeast mixture, add milk mixture and:
    1   (1)   egg, well beaten
    1½ cups   (375 mL)   all-purpose flour
    2 tsp.   (10 mL)   cinnamon
    1 tsp.   (5 mL)   allspice
    ½ tsp.   (2 mL)   cloves
    1   (1)   orange, grated rind of
    ½ cup   (125 mL)   unsweetened concentrated apple juice, warmed to 105-115°F (40-45°C)

Beat until smooth. Cover with a damp cloth. Let rise in a warm, 80-85°F (27-30°C), place until very light and bubbly, about 1¼ hours. Add and mix well:
    2 cups   (500 mL)   all-purpose flour
    ⅔ cup   (150 mL)   raisins

Turn out on a lightly floured board. Knead until smooth and elastic, about 10 minutes. Place dough in a greased mixing bowl; turn the dough over to grease the entire surface. Cover with a damp cloth. Let rise in a warm, 80-85°F (27-30°C), place until doubled in size, about 1 hour. Knead down; divide into egg-sized pieces; shape each piece into a ball; place on a greased baking sheet, about ½" (1.3 cm) apart. Cover and let rise until doubled, about 1 hour.

HOT CROSS BUNS (continued)

Beat until blended:
- 1 (1) egg yolk
- 1 tbsp. (15 mL) water

Brush egg mixture gently over the buns. With a sharp knife, cut a cross on top of each bun. Bake in the middle of the oven at 375°F (190°C) for about 25 minutes. Remove the buns from baking sheet; cool on wire rack. Makes 15 buns.

ROLLED CHEESEWICHES

Warm to 105-115°F (40-45°C):
- ½ cup (125 mL) unsweetened apple juice

Sprinkle with:
- 1 tbsp. (15 mL) active dry yeast (1 pkg.)

Let stand until surface is foamy, 10 minutes; stir with fork to moisten any dry particles.

Combine until dissolved:
- 3 tbsp. (45 mL) instant skim milk powder
- ½ cup (125 mL) hot water
- 2 tbsp. (30 mL) oil

Cool to 105-115°F (40-45°C). Add milk mixture to yeast mixture with:
- 1 (1) egg, beaten
- 1½ cups (375 mL) whole-wheat flour

Beat with a wooden spoon until smooth. Add and mix by hand:
- 1 cup (250 mL) unbleached OR all-purpose flour OR more to make a soft dough.

Turn out on a lightly floured board and knead until smooth and elastic, about 10 minutes. Place dough in a greased mixing bowl; turn dough over to grease entire surface. Cover with a damp cloth. Let rise in a warm, 80-85°F (27-30°C), place until doubled, about 1 hour. Divide dough in half. Roll out each half on a lightly floured board to 10" (25 cm) circle; cut each circle into 6 wedges. Spread each wedge with Cheese Filling, recipe follows, covering within ½" (1.3 cm) of edges. Starting at the curved side, roll each wedge to the point. Place on a lightly oiled baking sheet, point-side down. Cover and let rise in a warm place until doubled, about 50 minutes.

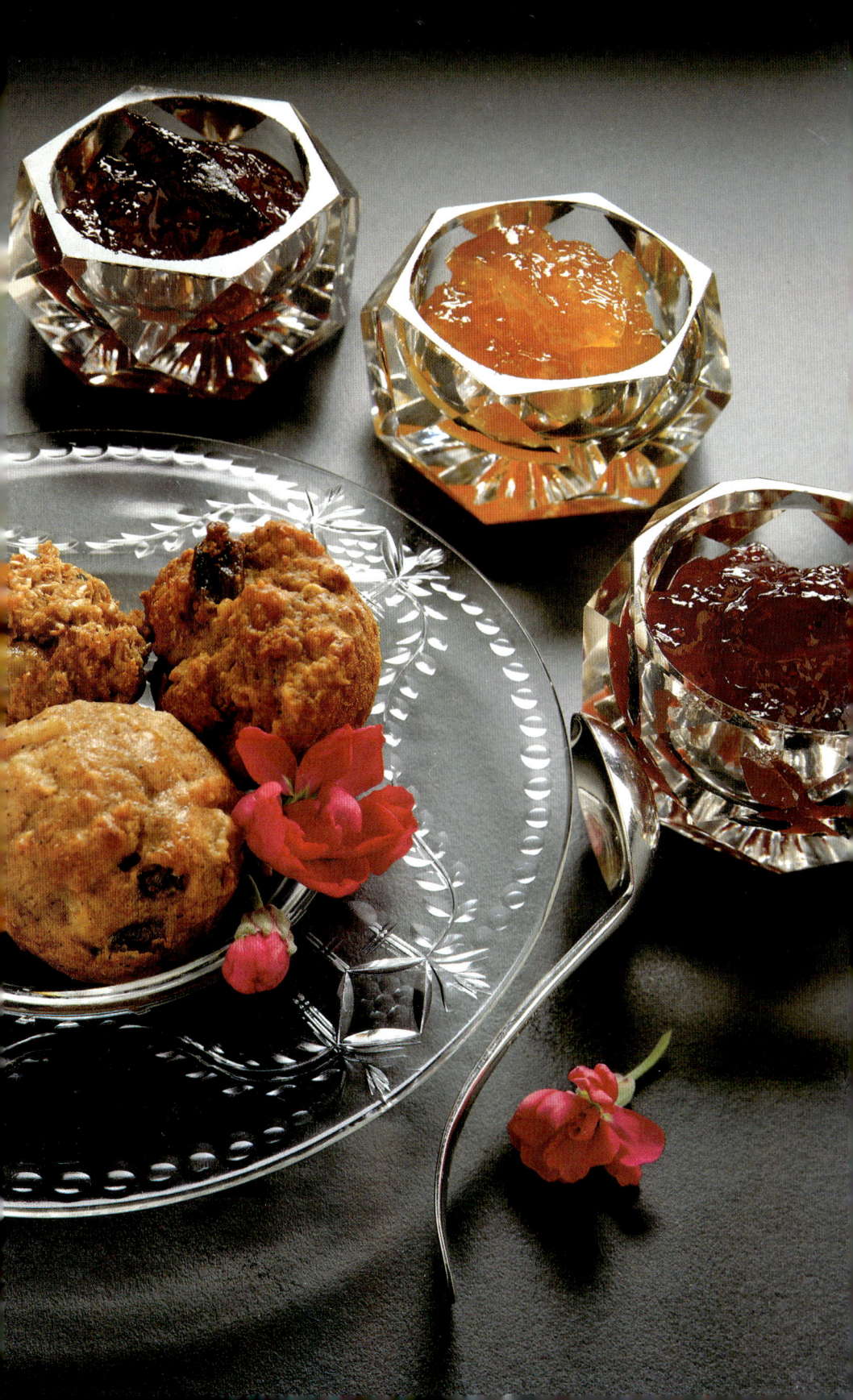

Plum Jam, page 59
Peach Jam, page 58
Rhubarb-Strawberry Jam, page 57
Banana-Nut-Bran Muffins, page 6
Oatmeal Muffins, page 6
Rice Raisin Muffins, page 7

ROLLED CHEESEWICHES (continued)

Beat together:
- 1 (1) egg white
- 2 tsp. (10 mL) water

Brush egg mixture gently over each roll. Bake in the middle of the oven at 375°F (190°C) until brown, 30-35 minutes. Makes 12.

CHEESE FILLING

Combine:
- 2 cups (500 mL) grated old Cheddar cheese
- 1 tsp. (5 mL) finely chopped onion
- ¼ tsp. (1 mL) pepper
- 1 (1) egg yolk, beaten

Divide filling into 12 equal portions; spread on wedges.

APRICOT LOG

Combine:
- ½ cup (125 mL) milk, scalded
- 2 tbsp. (30 mL) butter OR margarine
- ¼ tsp. (1 mL) salt

Cool to 105-115°F (40-45°C). In a mixing bowl, combine:
- 1 tbsp. (15 mL) unsweetened concentrated apple juice, defrosted
- 4 tbsp. (60 mL) hot water

Cool to 105-115°F (40-45°C). Sprinkle with:
- 1 tbsp. (15 mL) active dry yeast (1 pkg.)

Let stand until surface is foamy, 10 minutes; stir with fork to moisten any dry particles.

APRICOT LOG (continued)

Add milk mixture to yeast mixture and:
- 1 (1) egg, beaten
- 1½ cups (375 mL) all-purpose OR unbleached flour
- 3 tbsp. (45 mL) unsweetened concentrated apple juice, room temperature

Beat with a wooden spoon until smooth. Gradually mix in by hand:
- 1½ cups (375 mL) all-purpose OR unbleached flour

Turn out on lightly floured board; knead until smooth and elastic, 10 minutes. Place dough in a greased mixing bowl; turn over to grease entire surface. Cover bowl with a damp cloth. Let rise in a warm, 80-85°F (27-30°C), place until doubled, about 1 hour. Punch down dough; turn onto a lightly floured board; cover and let rest 10 minutes. Roll out to a 16" (40 cm) square; spread Apricot Filling, recipe follows, within ½" (1.3 cm) of the edges. Roll up dough jelly-roll fashion. Brush edge with:
- 1 (1) egg yolk, beaten

Press well to seal. Place on oiled baking sheet. Cover and let rise in a warm, 80-85°F (27-30°C), place until doubled, about 1 hour. Beat remainder of egg yolk with:
- 2 tsp. (10 mL) water

Brush roll with egg mixture. Bake in the middle of oven at 375°F (190°C) until brown, 35-40 minutes. Remove from pan. Makes 12 good-sized servings.

APRICOT FILLING

In a saucepan, combine:
- ½ lb. (250 g) finely sliced dried apricots
- ¾ cup (175 mL) unsweetened concentrated apple juice, defrosted
- 1 tbsp. (15 mL) lemon juice
- 4 tbsp. (60 mL) water

Bring to a boil, reduce to medium-low. Cook and stir until most of the liquid has been absorbed. Stir in; cool:
- ¾ cup (175 mL) toasted unsweetened shredded coconut

CHEESE PUFFS

Measure into a mixing bowl and cool to 105-115°F (40-45°C):
1 tbsp.	(	15 mL)	unsweetened concentrated apple juice, defrosted
3 tbsp.	(	45 mL)	boiling water

Sprinkle with:
1½ tsp.	(	7 mL)	active dry yeast (½ pkg.)

Let stand until foamy, about 10 minutes; stir with fork to moisten.

Combine until dissolved:
2 tbsp.	(	30 mL)	instant skim milk powder
4 tbsp.	(	60 mL)	hot water

To milk mixture, add and stir on low heat until melted:
4 tbsp.	(	60 mL)	butter OR margarine

Cool to 105-115°F (40-45°C). Add milk mixture to yeast mixture with:
1	(	1)	egg, beaten
⅔ cup	(	150 mL)	whole-wheat flour

Beat with an electric beater until smooth. Add:
1 tsp.	(	5 mL)	dry mustard
½ tsp.	(	2 mL)	paprika
⅛ tsp.	(	0.5 mL)	cayenne
2 tbsp.	(	30 mL)	unsweetened concentrated apple juice, room temperature
1 cup	(	250 mL)	grated old Cheddar cheese
⅓ cup	(	75 mL)	finely chopped onion
1 cup	(	250 mL)	all-purpose flour

Beat on low speed until blended. Cover with a damp cloth. Let rise in a warm, 80-85°F (27-30°C), place until doubled, about 1¼ hours. Stir down. Drop spoonfuls of batter, walnut-sized, onto an oiled baking sheet 1" (2.5 cm) apart. Cover, let rise in a warm place, until doubled, 1 hour.

Brush top with a mixture of:
1	(	1)	egg yolk
1 tbsp.	(	15 mL)	water

Bake in the middle of the oven at 375°F (190°C) until brown, 20-25 minutes. Remove puffs from baking sheet; cool on wire rack.

Makes 24 .

SEED AND GRAIN BREAD

In a large mixing bowl, combine:
- 6 tbsp. (90 mL) unsweetened concentrated apple juice, defrosted
- 2⅓ cups (575 mL) hot water

Cool to 105-115°F (40-45°C). Sprinkle with:
- 1 tbsp. (15 mL) active dry yeast (1 pkg.)

Let rise until foamy, about 10 minutes; stir with fork to moisten.

To yeast mixture, add:
- 4 tbsp. (60 mL) vegetable oil
- ½ tsp. (2 mL) salt
- 1 cup (250 mL) quick-cooking rolled oats
- 1 cup (250 mL) whole-wheat flour
- 1 cup (250 mL) all-purpose OR unbleached flour

Beat until smooth; cover bowl with a damp cloth. Let rise in a warm, 80-85°F (27-30°C), place until light and spongy, 1¼ hours.

Add and mix well:
- ¼ cup (60 mL) finely chopped walnuts
- 2 tbsp. (30 mL) flax seeds
- 2 tbsp. (30 mL) poppy seeds
- 2 tbsp. (30 mL) sesame seeds
- 2 tbsp. (30 mL) sunflower seeds
- 2 tbsp. (30 mL) millet
- ½ cup (125 mL) whole-wheat flour
- 2 cups (500 mL) all-purpose OR unbleached flour

Turn out onto a floured board. Knead until smooth and elastic, 15 minutes. Place in a large greased bowl. Turn dough over to grease entire surface. Cover with a damp cloth; and let rise in a warm, 80-85°F (27-30°C), place until doubled, about 1 hour. Knead down; divide in half; shape into loaves. Place in 2 oiled loaf pans, 8½"x4½" (21x11 cm). Cover; let rise in a warm place until doubled, about 1 hour.

Beat until blended:
- 1 (1) egg yolk
- 2 tsp. (10 mL) water

Brush egg mixture over loaves. Bake in the middle of the oven at 350°F (180°C) for 1 hour. Remove from pan; cool on wire rack. Makes 2 loaves.

Salad and Fruit Dressings

FRENCH DRESSING

Measure into a small jar with a tight fitting lid and shake thoroughly:

6 tbsp.	(	90 mL)	salad oil
2 tbsp.	(	30 mL)	vinegar
1 tsp.	(	5 mL)	unsweetened concentrated apple juice, defrosted
⅛ tsp.	(	0.5 mL)	dry mustard
⅛ tsp.	(	0.5 mL)	paprika
			dash of pepper

Refrigerate. Shake well before using. Makes ½ cup (125 mL).

SOUR CREAM DRESSING

Stir until blended:

1 cup	(	250 mL)	sour cream, 5.5% m.f.
3 tbsp.	(	45 mL)	vinegar
1 tsp.	(	5 mL)	unsweetened concentrated apple juice, defrosted
½ tsp.	(	2 mL)	paprika
¼ tsp.	(	1 mL)	salt
			pinch of cayenne

Refrigerate. Serve with baked potato, lettuce or vegetable salad. Makes about 1¼ cups (300 mL).

LOW-CALORIE MAYONNAISE

Blend until smooth:
1 cup	(	250 mL)	cottage cheese, 1% m.f.
2 tsp.	(	10 mL)	salad oil
4 tsp.	(	20 mL)	vinegar OR lemon juice
2 tsp.	(	10 mL)	unsweetened concentrated apple juice, defrosted
¼-½ tsp.	(	1-2 mL)	dry mustard, according to taste
			pinch of cayenne

Refrigerate. Makes 1 cup (250 mL).

THOUSAND ISLAND DRESSING

Prepare Low-Calorie Mayonnaise, see above, and add:
4 tbsp.	(	60 mL)	Ketchup, page 46, 47
1 tbsp.	(	15 mL)	chopped green pepper
1 tbsp.	(	15 mL)	minced onion
1 tbsp.	(	15 mL)	minced stuffed olives
1	(	1)	chopped hard-cooked egg

Stir well; refrigerate. Makes about 1½ cups (375 mL).

SOUR CREAM HORSERADISH DRESSING

Stir until blended:
1 cup	(	250 mL)	sour cream, 5.5% m.f.
1 tbsp.	(	15 mL)	prepared horseradish
1 tsp.	(	5 mL)	unsweetened concentrated apple juice, defrosted
¼ tsp.	(	1 mL)	dry mustard
¼ tsp.	(	1 mL)	paprika
¼ tsp.	(	1 mL)	salt

Refrigerate. Serve with fish, roast or any cold meats. Makes 1 cup (250 mL).

COOKED SALAD DRESSING

Combine in top of double boiler:

1 tbsp.	(	15 mL)	cornstarch
1 tsp.	(	5 mL)	dry mustard
⅛ tsp.	(	0.5 mL)	paprika
¼ tsp.	(	1 mL)	salt
2 tbsp.	(	30 mL)	unsweetened concentrated apple juice, defrosted

Add and beat with a wire whip until blended:

| ⅔ cup | (| 150 mL) | milk |
| 2 | (| 2) | egg yolks |

Stir in:

| ⅓ cup | (| 75 mL) | vinegar |

Cook and stir over boiling water until thickened. Cover and cook 5 minutes longer. Cool. Pour into jar. Cover. Refrigerate. Makes 1 cup (250 mL).

COTTAGE CHEESE HORSERADISH DRESSING

Blend until smooth:

½ cup	(	125 mL)	cottage cheese, 1% m.f.
2 tbsp.	(	30 mL)	milk
1 tsp.	(	5 mL)	vinegar
1 tsp.	(	5 mL)	unsweetened concentrated apple juice, defrosted
1 tsp.	(	5 mL)	prepared horseradish
			pinch of cayenne

Serve with roast beef, cold cuts, etc. Makes ⅔ cup (150 mL).

COTTAGE CHEESE FRUIT DRESSING

Blend in a blender until smooth:
- 1 cup (250 mL) cottage cheese, 1% m.f.
- 1 tbsp. (15 mL) milk
- 3 tbsp. (45 mL) unsweetened concentrated apple juice, defrosted
- 2 tsp. (10 mL) lemon juice

Serve as topping on fruit salad, stewed fruit, applesauce, etc. Makes 1¼ cups (300 mL).

WHIPPED CREAM FRUIT SALAD DRESSING

Combine in top of double boiler:
- 2½ tsp. (12 mL) cornstarch
- 4½ tbsp. (68 mL) unsweetened concentrated pineapple OR apple juice, defrosted
- 1½ tbsp. (23 mL) lemon juice
- 6 tbsp. (90 mL) water

Cook and stir over boiling water until thick and clear.

Beat:
- 1 (1) egg OR 2 egg yolks

Stir half of the hot mixture into egg or yolks, mix well, return to hot mixture, cook and stir 3 minutes. Refrigerate until cold.

Whip until stiff:
- ⅓ cup (75 mL) whipping cream

Fold into cold mixture. Makes 1 cup (250 mL).

Vegetables

COLESLAW

Combine in a large bowl:
- 3 cups (750 mL) finely shredded cabbage
- 1 (1) medium carrot, grated
- 1 (1) small onion, thinly sliced
- ½ cup (125 mL) thinly sliced celery

Mix together:
- ⅓ cup (75 mL) vinegar
- 2 tbsp. (30 mL) salad oil
- 3 tbsp. (45 mL) unsweetened concentrated apple juice, defrosted
- ½ tsp. (2 mL) dry mustard
- ¼ tsp. (1 mL) pepper
- 1 tsp. (5 mL) celery seed

Pour mixture over vegetables; toss lightly until blended. Refrigerate. Serves 4-6.

APPLE COLESLAW

Combine:
- 2 cups (500 mL) finely shredded cabbage
- 1 (1) medium apple, peeled, cut into strips
- 1 tbsp. (15 mL) lemon juice OR vinegar
- ½ cup (125 mL) grated Cheddar cheese

Combine:
- ½ cup (125 mL) plain yogurt
- 4 tsp. (20 mL) unsweetened concentrated apple juice, defrosted
- 2 tbsp. (30 mL) vinegar
- ⅛ tsp. (0.5 mL) dry mustard
- pinch of cayenne

Pour yogurt mixture over cabbage; toss lightly. Refrigerate. Serves 2-4.

POTATO SALAD

Cook in their jackets until tender, about 20-30 minutes:
- 1½ lbs. (750 g) potatoes, scrubbed (about 5 medium)
- boiling water to cover

Combine in a large bowl:
- ½ cup (125 mL) diagonally sliced celery
- ¼ cup (60 mL) grated carrots
- ⅓ cup (75 mL) finely chopped onions
- 2 (2) hard-cooked eggs, chopped

Peel the cooked potatoes; cut into cubes; add to vegetable mixture.

Blend until smooth:
- 1½ cups (375 mL) cottage cheese, 1% m.f.
- 1 tbsp. (15 mL) salad oil
- 5 tbsp. (75 mL) vinegar OR lemon juice
- 4 tsp. (20 mL) unsweetened concentrated apple juice, defrosted
- ½ tsp. (2 mL) dry mustard
- ¼ tsp. (1 mL) paprika
- 1 (1) garlic clove, minced (optional)
- ½ tsp. (2 mL) salt
- ½ tsp. (2 mL) pepper

Pour dressing over potato mixture. Mix gently with a wooden spoon. Cover and refrigerate 2 hours. Before serving, toss with:
- 2 tbsp. (30 mL) chopped parsley

Serves 6.

TO STORE GARLIC

Store garlic in a paper bag in a cool, dark, dry place on the kitchen shelf. It should keep several months. Garlic may be stored in refrigerator for a short time, but it will become mouldy if left for a long time.

SPICY RED CABBAGE

Cut into 4 sections; remove core and finely slice:
    1 (1) medium red cabbage, about 2 lbs. (1 kg)

Wash cabbage in warm water, drain, place in a pot with:
    1 cup (250 mL) water

Sauté and drain off fat:
    ¼ lb. (115 g) bacon slices, chopped

Add:
    1 (1) large onion, peeled, thinly sliced

Sauté onion until lightly browned; add to cabbage with:
    6 (6) whole allspice
    6 (6) juniper berries
    2 (2) bay leaves
    ½ tsp. (2 mL) salt

Bring cabbage mixture to a boil, then simmer, covered, for 40 minutes, stirring occasionally. Uncover. Cook on high heat, stirring often, until all liquid is absorbed. Add; stir to mix:
    2 (2) cooking apples, peeled, cored and thinly sliced
    ⅓ cup (75 mL) unsweetened concentrated apple juice, defrosted
    ⅓ cup (75 mL) vinegar

Cook, stirring occasionally, until apples are tender and most of the liquid has been absorbed. Adjust seasoning according to taste. Serves 6-8.

See photograph on page 32A.

SWEET AND SOUR RED CABBAGE

Cut into 4 sections; remove core; finely shred:
    1 (1) medium red cabbage, about 2 lbs. (1 kg)

Wash cabbage in warm water; drain; place in a pot with:
    1 cup (250 mL) water

Heat in a skillet:
    1 tbsp. (15 mL) butter, margarine OR cooking oil

Add:
    1 (1) large onion, peeled, thinly sliced

Sauté onion until a light brown; add to cabbage. Bring to a boil, then simmer, covered, for 40 minutes, stirring occasionally. Uncover. Cook on high heat, stirring often, until all liquid is absorbed. Add; stir to mix:

    2 (2) cooking apples, peeled, cored and thinly sliced
    6 tbsp. (90 mL) unsweetened concentrated apple juice, defrosted
    ½ cup (125 mL) vinegar
    1 tsp. (5 mL) salt
    ⅛ tsp. (0.5 mL) cloves

Cover and cook 10 minutes, stirring occasionally.

Combine until smooth:
    2 tsp. (10 mL) cornstarch
    1 tbsp. (15 mL) water

Stir cornstarch mixture into hot mixture. Cook and stir until it thickens and boils. Boil 1 minute. Serves 6-8.

SWEET AND SOUR BEANS

Remove ends and strings; cut into 2" (5 cm) lengths:
- 1 lb. (500 g) green beans

Wash beans and place in a saucepan; add:
- boiling water to almost cover beans

Cover and cook until tender, 20-25 minutes. Turn off heat.

Skim cooked beans into a bowl; set aside. To liquid in saucepan add:
- 2 tbsp. (30 mL) unsweetened concentrated apple juice, defrosted
- 4 tbsp. (60 mL) vinegar (OR more to taste)
- 1 tbsp. (15 mL) cornstarch

Mix until cornstarch has dissolved. Add:
- 1 (1) small onion, thinly sliced crosswise

Cook and stir over low heat until thick and clear. Add cooked beans; mix well. Heat until hot and serve. Serves 4.

BAKED TURNIPS

Mix well:
- 4 cups (1 L) mashed turnips, page 30
- 1 tbsp. (15 mL) unsweetened concentrated apple juice, defrosted
- 1/8 tsp. (0.5 mL) paprika
- salt and pepper to taste

Beat until stiff and set aside:
- 2 (2) egg whites

Beat:
- 2 (2) egg yolks

Add yolks to turnip; blend well. Fold in egg whites. Pour into an oiled 6-cup (1.5 L) baking dish. Bake at 375°F (190°C) for 30 minutes. Serves 6.

MASHED TURNIPS

Peel and wash:
    1 (1)   medium turnip, about 2 lbs. (1 kg)

Slice or dice turnip into a saucepan.

Add (optional):
    1 (1)   medium carrot, scraped, washed, sliced

Cover with:
    boiling water

Cook in rapidly boiling water until tender, 20-25 minutes. Drain. Mash turnips in the saucepan. Place over low heat 5-10 minutes to dry turnips, stirring constantly. Add:
    1 tsp. (5 mL)   unsweetened concentrated apple juice, defrosted

Season according to taste with:
    salt and pepper

Makes about 4 cups (1 L).

See photograph on page 32A.

GLAZED SQUASH

Wash and cut into quarters:
    1 (1)   medium pepper squash

Scrape out seeds. Pierce pulp with a two-tined fork in 4 or 5 places.

Spread each squash quarter with:
    1 tsp. (5 mL)   butter OR margarine
    1 tbsp. (15 mL)   unsweetened concentrated apple juice, defrosted

Arrange squash cut-side up in a shallow pan. Add:
    3 tbsp. (45 mL)   hot water

Cover with foil and bake at 400°F (200°C) until tender, about 30 minutes. Serves 4.

GLAZED CARROTS

In a saucepan, combine:
- 2 cups (500 mL) **diagonally sliced carrots**
- ⅔ cup (150 mL) **boiling water**

Bring to a boil, reduce heat to medium-low, cover and cook until carrots are tender, about 20-25 minutes.

Mix until smooth:
- 2 tsp. (10 mL) **cornstarch**
- 2 tbsp. (30 mL) **unsweetened concentrated apple juice, defrosted**

Stir cornstarch mixture into hot mixture. Cook and stir over low heat until thick. Serves 4.

HARVARD BEETS

Combine in top of double boiler:
- 2 tsp. (10 mL) **cornstarch**
- 4 tbsp. (60 mL) **unsweetened concentrated apple juice, defrosted**
- 4 tbsp. (60 mL) **vinegar**
- 3 tbsp. (45 mL) **water**
- 4 (4) **whole cloves**

Cook and stir over boiling water until thick and smooth. Add:
- 3 cups (750 mL) **diced OR sliced cooked beets**

Mix well; cover; allow to stand over hot water until ready to serve. Serves 5-6.

Main Dishes

BEEF TOMATO

Slice across the grain into thin strips:
- 1½ lbs. (750 g) sirloin steak

Combine the beef and:
- 1 tbsp. (15 mL) soy sauce
- 1 tbsp. (15 mL) vegetable oil
- ¼ tsp. (1 mL) pepper
- ½ tsp. (2 mL) sesame oil, toasted

Marinate for about 1 hour.

Drain 6 tbsp. (90 mL) of juice from:
- 28 oz. (796 mL) can tomatoes

Cut whole tomatoes into 4 quarters.

Prepare:
- 1 (1) small onion, peeled and sliced
- 1 tbsp. (15 mL) peeled, minced ginger root
- 1 (1) garlic clove, minced

Heat in a large frying pan or wok until it smokes:
- 2 tbsp. (30 mL) oil

Sprinkle with:
- a little salt

Add the sliced beef; stir-fry until it is no longer red; set aside. Add the onion, minced ginger root and garlic. Stir-fry 30 seconds. Add tomatoes and remaining juice. Cover and cook over medium heat 7 minutes. Add beef. Cook and stir until heated through.

Combine the 6 tbsp. (90 mL) of juice and:
- 2½ tbsp. (38 mL) cornstarch
- 3 tbsp. (45 mL) vinegar
- 1 tsp. (5 mL) unsweetened concentrated apple juice, defrosted

Add to hot liquid. Cook and stir until it thickens and boils. Stir-fry to coat vegetables and beef with sauce. Serve with rice. Serves 4.

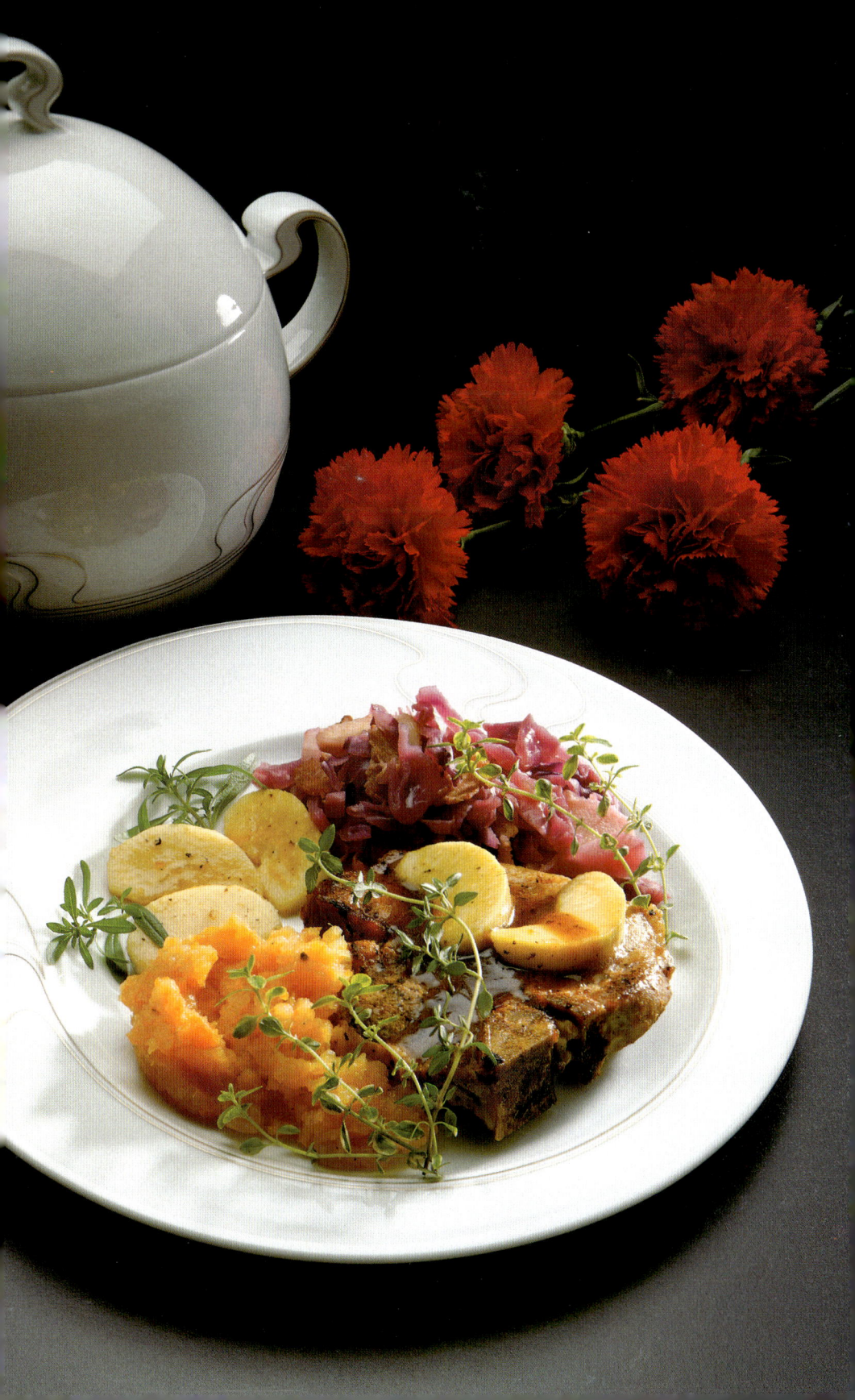

Apple Pork Chops, page 39
Tangy Apple Wedges, page 38
Mashed Turnips, page 30
Spicy Red Cabbage, page 27

SAUERBRATEN

Place in a large bowl:
3 lbs.	(	1.5 kg)	beef blade, chuck, rump, shoulder OR brisket

Add:
1 cup	(	250 mL)	vinegar
4 tbsp.	(	60 mL)	unsweetened concentrated apple juice, defrosted
2¾ cups	(	675 mL)	boiling water
1	(	1)	large onion, peeled and sliced
2	(	2)	bay leaves
8	(	8)	peppercorns
3	(	3)	whole cloves

Cover; marinate in refrigerator for 24 hours to a maximum of 4 days; turn meat several times. Drain and reserve marinade. In a heavy saucepan, heat on high:

2 tbsp.	(	30 mL)	cooking oil

Add meat, brown on all sides. Add marinade. Cover; bring to a boil; reduce heat and simmer until tender, 2½-3 hours. Turn meat several times during cooking. Remove meat to a heated platter. Pour off liquid; skim and discard excess fat. Serve marinade as is or thicken with flour by combining:

2⅓ cups	(	575 mL)	hot marinade
½ tsp.	(	2 mL)	soy sauce
3 tbsp.	(	45 mL)	flour

Return marinade to saucepan. Bring to a boil; cook and stir 2 minutes. Serve with meat. Serves 6.

BEEF PIZZA

Heat in a saucepan:
    1 tbsp.   (15 mL)   cooking oil

Add:
       1 lb.   (500 g)   lean ground beef
       1   (1)   small onion, peeled, finely chopped

Break up beef; sauté 5 minutes.

Add:
      28 oz.   (796 mL)   can tomatoes, drained and crushed
      1   (1)   small green pepper, seeded, chopped
      2 tsp.   (10 mL)   unsweetened concentrated apple juice, defrosted
      1   (1)   garlic clove, minced
      ½ tsp.   (2 mL)   salt
      ¼ tsp.   (1 mL)   pepper

Cover beef mixture and simmer 10 minutes. Turn off heat. Keep warm until Pizza Crust, recipe follows, has been baked 10 minutes at 375°F (190°C). Remove crust from oven. Spread hot beef mixture evenly over crust. Sprinkle with:
      4 oz.   (115 g)   Gruyère cheese, grated
                                   dried oregano

Bake at 375°F (190°C) until pizza edges are lightly browned, about 25 minutes. Serves 8.

WHOLE-WHEAT PIZZA CRUST

Combine:
    1 cup   (250 mL)   whole-wheat flour
    1 tbsp.   (15 mL)   baking powder

Mix in with a fork:
    2 tbsp.   (30 mL)   oil

Beat together:
    1   (1)   egg
    5 tsp.   (25 mL)   water

PIZZA CRUST (continued)

Stir into flour mixture. Press dough firmly into a ball. Roll out on a lightly floured board to fit an oiled 12" (30 cm) pizza pan, building up edges slightly to hold filling. Prick all over with fork. Bake at 375°F (190°C) for 10 minutes. Remove from oven. Spread topping evenly on prebaked crust. Return to oven; bake until edges of pizza are light brown. Makes one 12" (30 cm) crust.

HAWAIIAN MEATBALLS

Mix with a fork until blended:
1½ lbs.	(	750 g)	ground chuck OR ground round steak
1	(	1)	small onion, peeled, finely chopped
1	(	1)	egg, beaten
1 tsp.	(	5 mL)	horseradish (optional)
1 tsp.	(	5 mL)	soy sauce
1	(	1)	garlic clove, minced
½ tsp.	(	2 mL)	pepper

Shape meat mixture into ¾" (1.9 cm) meatballs. Heat in a large frying pan or wok:
1 tbsp.	(	15 mL)	cooking oil

Add meatballs and brown on all sides. Remove meatballs and discard fat. Place in frying pan or wok:
1	(	1)	green pepper, seeded and sliced
19 oz.	(	540 mL)	can unsweetened pineapple chunks, undrained

Cover and simmer 5 minutes. Add meatballs and:
4 tbsp.	(	60 mL)	unsweetened concentrated apple juice, defrosted.
1 tbsp.	(	15 mL)	soy sauce

Cook and stir until the meatballs are heated through. Blend until smooth:
2 tbsp.	(	30 mL)	cornstarch
4 tbsp.	(	60 mL)	vinegar

Stir cornstarch mixture into the hot liquid. Cook and stir until it thickens and boils. Boil 1 minute. Serves 4-6.

CABBAGE ROLLS

Discard withered outer leaves and cut off the base of:
    1 (1)   **large cabbage**

Remove the coarser leaves but save them to line frying pan. Cut out the core; run water from tap into hole to loosen leaves. Gently remove 8 leaves; place them in boiling water and parboil 8 minutes; drain; trim off the thick centre vein of each leaf.

If leaves are difficult to remove, place the whole cabbage, right side up, in about 2" (5 cm) of boiling water for 3-5 minutes; remove loosened leaves; repeat until enough leaves have been removed.

Combine thoroughly and divide into 8 portions:

1 lb.	(500 g)	**ground meat (beef, veal, pork, chicken, etc.)**
⅓ cup	(75 mL)	**long-grain rice, uncooked**
1	(1)	**small onion, peeled and chopped**
1	(1)	**egg, beaten**
1	(1)	**garlic clove, minced**
½ tsp.	(2 mL)	**salt**
¼ tsp.	(1 mL)	**pepper**

Place each portion in the centre of a cabbage leaf, fold over sides and roll up. Place rolls, seam side down, in a large frying pan lined with washed coarser cabbage leaves.

Over cabbage rolls, pour:
    2½ cups   (625 mL)   **tomato juice**

Bring to a boil, cover and cook over medium heat for 10 minutes. Reduce heat to medium-low, cover and cook until cabbage leaves are tender, about 50 minutes, basting occasionally. Spoon off some liquid from pan and mix with:

3 tbsp.	(45 mL)	**unsweetened concentrated apple juice, defrosted**
3 tbsp.	(45 mL)	**vinegar**

Return vinegar mixture to pan and baste cabbage rolls with it. Adjust seasoning, as desired. Serves 4.

CURRIED LAMB

Trim; cut into 1" (2.5 cm) cubes:
2 lbs. (**1 kg)** boneless lamb shoulder

Heat:
2 tbsp. (**30 mL)** oil

Add lamb; brown on all sides. Add:
1 cup (**250 mL)** water

Bring lamb to a boil; reduce to medium-low. Cover and simmer 45 minutes.

Add:

1	(	**1)**	medium onion, peeled and sliced
2	(	**2)**	medium apples, peeled, cored and sliced
1	(	**1)**	celery stalk, sliced diagonally
1½ tbsp.	(	**22 mL)**	curry powder
2 tsp.	(	**10 mL)**	unsweetened concentrated apple juice, defrosted
1 tsp.	(	**5 mL)**	soy sauce
½ tsp.	(	**2 mL)**	salt
1 tbsp.	(	**15 mL)**	peeled, minced ginger root
¼ tsp.	(	**1 mL)**	pepper

Cover and continue to cook until meat is tender, about 15 minutes longer.

Combine until smooth:
3 tbsp. (**45 mL)** all-purpose flour
½ cup (**125 mL)** milk

Add milk mixture to hot liquid. Cook and stir over medium heat until the sauce thickens and bubbles. Combine lamb mixture with the sauce; cook and stir until heated through. Serve with rice. Serves 4.

BAKED BEANS

Wash; discarding beans that float:
    1½ cups (375 mL)   dried beans (navy OR any other)

Soak overnight in:
    4 cups (1 L)   water

Bring beans slowly to a boil; cover and simmer until tender, about 30 minutes. Preheat oven to 250°F (125°C).

Spread on the bottom of a beanpot or casserole with a cover:
    1 (1)   small onion, peeled, chopped

Spoon the beans and liquid over the onion.

Mix together:
    3 tbsp. (45 mL)   unsweetened concentrated apple juice, defrosted
    3 tbsp. (45 mL)   Ketchup, page 46, 47
    1 tsp. (5 mL)   dry mustard
    ½ tsp. (2 mL)   salt
    ¼ tsp. (1 mL)   pepper

Pour ketchup mixture over the beans. Top with:
    ¼ lb. (125 g)   salt pork, sliced

Cover and bake 5 hours. Uncover and bake ½ hour longer. Serves 4.

TANGY APPLE WEDGES

Combine in a small saucepan:
    4 tbsp. (60 mL)   vinegar
    5 tbsp. (75 mL)   unsweetened concentrated apple juice, defrosted
    1 tbsp. (15 mL)   water
    1 (1)   cinnamon stick

Peel, core and cut into quarters:
    3 (3)   firm apples

Cut each quarter into 3 wedges. Bring the vinegar mixture to a boil; reduce to medium low. Add apple wedges, a few at a time. Cook, stirring a little, until a fork can pierce easily into an apple wedge (but apples are not soft), about 3 minutes. Serves 6.

See photograph on page 32A.

APPLE PORK CHOPS

In a large heavy frying pan, heat on high:
- **2 tbsp.   (30 mL)   oil**

Add:
- **6   (6)   loin pork chops, ¾" (1.9 cm) thick**

Lightly brown chops on both sides. Add:
- **⅔ cup   (150 mL)   unsweetened concentrated apple juice, defrosted**
- **1 cup   (250 mL)   hot water**
- **½ tsp.   (2 mL)   salt**
- **¼ tsp.   (1 mL)   pepper**

Bring to a boil; reduce to medium-low. Cover and simmer until tender, 45-55 minutes. Transfer chops to a heated platter.

Combine until smooth:
- **2 tbsp.   (30 mL)   cornstarch**
- **1 tbsp.   (15 mL)   lemon juice**
- **4 tbsp.   (60 mL)   water**

Stir cornstarch mixture into hot apple liquid. Cook and stir until it thickens and boils. Boil and stir 1 minute. Pour over chops. Serve with Tangy Apple Wedges, page 38. Serves 6.

See photograph on page 32A.

PINEAPPLE-GLAZED HAM

Place skin side up on wire rack in a shallow uncovered baking pan:
- **1   (1)   cooked ham**

Bake 15 minutes per pound at 325°F (160°C); 30 minutes before end of baking time, remove ham from oven. Cut off rind (skin), leaving a thin layer of fat. Cut criss-cross slashes, about 1" (2.5 cm) apart, through the fat to the meat. Where criss-crosses intersect, insert:
- **whole cloves**

With toothpicks, fasten along top of ham:
- **slices of unsweetened pineapple**

Spoon about ⅓ of Pineapple Glaze, page 40, over ham. Return ham to oven; bake 30-40 minutes, basting with glaze every 10 minutes. Let stand 15 minutes before carving.

PINEAPPLE GLAZE

Combine until dissolved:
- 5 tsp. (25 mL) cornstarch
- ¾ cup (175 mL) juice from canned pineapple
- ⅔ cup (150 mL) unsweetened concentrated pineapple juice, defrosted

Cook and stir until glaze thickens and boils. Boil and stir 1 minute. Makes about 1⅓ cups (325 mL).

BARBECUED SPARERIBS

In a large saucepan, place:
- 4 lbs. (1.8 kg) pork spareribs
- 1 tsp. (5 mL) salt
- water to cover spareribs

Bring to a rolling boil, reduce heat and simmer until tender, 50-60 minutes. Drain. Place ribs in a shallow pan and baste them with Barbecue Sauce, recipe follows. Set the pan on the broiler rack 5" (13 cm) from heat. Broil about 7 minutes. Turn; baste other side with Barbecue Sauce and broil another 7 minutes. Serve immediately. Serves 4.

BARBECUE SAUCE

In a small saucepan, combine:
- 1 cup (250 mL) Ketchup, pages 46, 47
- 3 tbsp. (45 mL) unsweetened concentrated apple juice, defrosted
- 3 tbsp. (45 mL) vinegar
- 1 tsp. (5 mL) soy sauce
- ½ tsp. (2 mL) dry mustard
- 1 (1) garlic clove, minced

Bring to a boil. Simmer and stir 5 minutes.

SWEET AND SOUR SPARERIBS

In a large saucepan, add:
- 4 lbs. (1.8 kg) pork spareribs
- 1 tsp. (5 mL) salt
- water to cover spareribs

Bring to a rolling boil; reduce heat. Cover and simmer until tender, 50-60 minutes. Drain. Cut into one-rib pieces. Place ribs on a preheated platter. Pour over ribs:

Sweet and Sour Sauce OR
Sweet and Sour Pineapple Sauce

Serves 4-6.

SWEET AND SOUR SAUCE

In a small saucepan, combine:
- 3 tbsp. (45 mL) cornstarch
- 1 (1) garlic clove, minced
- ½ tsp. (2 mL) salt
- ⅛ tsp. (0.5 mL) cayenne
- ½ cup (125 mL) unsweetened concentrated apple juice, defrosted
- ½ cup (125 mL) vinegar
- 2½ cups (625 mL) water

Simmer and stir until mixture thickens and boils. Boil and stir 1 minute.

SWEET AND SOUR PINEAPPLE SAUCE

Drain well:
- 14 oz. (398 mL) unsweetened pineapple chunks

Prepare Sweet and Sour Sauce and add drained pineapple chunks.

LEMON CHICKEN

Skin, bone and cut into bite-sized pieces:
  2 (2) whole (double) chicken breasts

In a plastic bag mix together:
  ¼ cup (60 mL) all-purpose flour
  ¼ tsp. (1 mL) grated lemon rind
  ½ tsp. (2 mL) minced garlic
  ½ tsp. (2 mL) salt
  ¼ tsp. (1 mL) pepper

Add chicken pieces; shake until all pieces are coated. Heat in a large frying pan or wok:
  2 tbsp. (30 mL) cooking oil

Add chicken pieces; stir-fry until chicken is cooked through, 10-15 minutes. Combine:
  ¼ cup (60 mL) lemon juice
  ¾ cup (175 mL) chicken stock OR water
  2 tbsp. (30 mL) unsweetened concentrated apple juice, defrosted
  2 tsp. (10 mL) soy sauce
  ¼ tsp. (1 mL) grated lemon rind

Pour over chicken. Bring to a boil; stir and cook 2 minutes. Serve immediately. Serves 4.

PINEAPPLE CHICKEN

Skin, and bone and cut into bite-sized pieces:
  2 (2) whole (double) chicken breasts

Sprinkle over chicken pieces:
  1 tsp. (5 mL) peeled, minced ginger root
  1 (1) garlic clove, minced
  ¼ tsp. (1 mL) pepper
  1 tbsp. (15 mL) cornstarch
  1 tbsp. (15 mL) soy sauce

Mix well. Set aside for 4 hours. Place in a large frying pan or wok. Add:
  14 oz. (398 mL) can unsweetened pineapple chunks, undrained
  5 tbsp. (75 mL) vinegar

PINEAPPLE CHICKEN (continued)

Mix pineapple and chicken well. Bring to a boil, cover and cook until chicken is cooked through, 10-15 minutes. Combine until dissolved:

2 tbsp.	(	30 mL)	cornstarch
4 tbsp.	(	60 mL)	unsweetened concentrated apple juice, defrosted
2 tbsp.	(	30 mL)	water

Stir cornstarch mixture into hot mixture. Cook and stir until thickened. Boil 1 minute. Adjust seasoning to taste. Serves 4.

ORANGE BARBECUED CHICKEN

In a large saucepan, bring to a rolling boil for 5 minutes:

8	(	8)	large chicken legs (drumsticks and thighs attached)
1	(	1)	bay leaf
1	(	1)	garlic clove, minced
½ tsp.	(	2 mL)	salt
¼ tsp.	(	1 mL)	pepper
			water to cover chicken legs

Reduce heat, cover, simmer until tender, about 50-60 minutes. Turn off heat; cool to room temperature. Refrigerate liquid (stock) for future use. If desired, remove skin from chicken legs. Arrange legs in a single layer in a shallow pan. Brush with Orange Barbecue Sauce. Set the pan on broiler rack, 5" (13 cm) from heat. Broil 7 minutes. Turn, brush with sauce and broil about 7 minutes. Serves 4-8.

ORANGE BARBECUE SAUCE

In a small saucepan, combine:

4 tsp.	(	20 mL)	cornstarch
½ tsp.	(	2 mL)	minced garlic
½ cup	(	125 mL)	unsweetened concentrated orange juice, defrosted
⅔ cup	(	150 mL)	water
2 tbsp.	(	30 mL)	soy sauce
1 tbsp.	(	15 mL)	lemon juice

Cook and stir until sauce thickens and boils. Boil and stir 1 minute.

ROAST DUCK À L'ORANGE

Preheat oven to 450°F (230°C). Wash; dry well:
 4-5 lbs.   (1.8-2.3 kg)   duck, ready to cook

Tie wings and legs to body. Place duck breast-side up on a wire rack in a shallow roasting pan. Put in oven, uncovered; reduce heat to 325°F (160°C) immediately. After baking 25 minutes, prick skin all over with a fork, to release fat; repeat 3 or 4 times. Turn duck over, halfway through baking. Bake until tender and duck is nicely browned, about 3 hours.

To serve, cut up the duck; arrange on a preheated platter. Pour Orange Sauce, page 60, over duck.

Garnish with 8 thin unpeeled orange slices, cut crosswise. Cilantro (Chinese or Italian parsley) or fresh thyme sprigs also make an attractive garnish. Serves 4.

SWEET AND SOUR FISH

Thaw, if frozen, just until it can be cut readily into individual serving portions:
 2 lbs.   (1 kg)   turbot, haddock, OR other fish fillets

Combine in a large frying pan or wok:
 ½ cup   (125 mL)   tomato juice
 ⅓ cup   (75 mL)   unsweetened concentrated apple juice, defrosted
 ⅓ cup   (75 mL)   vinegar
 2 tsp.   (10 mL)   soy sauce
 ¼ tsp.   (1 mL)   paprika

Add fish fillets. Bring to a boil; reduce to medium-low. Cover and simmer until fork pierces easily through fish, 10 minutes per 1" (2.5 cm) thickness for fresh fish, double the time for frozen fillets. Remove fish to preheated platter.

Combine:
 2 tbsp. (30 mL)   cornstarch
 2 tbsp. (30 mL)   water

Stir cornstarch mixture into hot juice mixture. Cook and stir until sauce thickens and boils. Boil and stir 1 minute longer. Pour over fish. Serves 4-6.

TUNA PIZZA

PIZZA CRUST

Oil a 12" (30 cm) pizza pan.

Combine:
½ tsp.	(	2 mL)	unsweetened concentrated apple juice, defrosted
⅔ cup	(	150 mL)	water at 105-115°F (40-45°C)

Sprinkle with:
1 tbsp.	(	15 mL)	active dry yeast (1 pkg.)

Let stand until surface is foamy, 10 minutes; stir with fork to moisten any dry particles.

Measure into a mixing bowl:
1½ cups	(	375 mL)	all-purpose flour
¼ tsp.	(	1 mL)	salt

To flour add yeast liquid and:
2 tbsp.	(	30 mL)	oil

Stir to make dough. Turn out on a lightly floured board and knead 10 minutes. Roll out dough to fit prepared pan. Transfer to pan; build up edges slightly to hold topping. Prick dough all over with a fork. Spread with Tuna Topping, recipe follows. Let stand 10 minutes. Bake at 400°F (200°C) until edges are lightly browned, about 25 minutes. Serves 8.

TUNA TOPPING

Cover pizza crust with the following, in the order given:
10 oz.	(	250 g)	mozzarella cheese, sliced
1¼ lbs.	(	625 g)	tomatoes, peeled, sliced
1	(	1)	small onion, peeled and chopped
6.5 oz.	(	184 g)	tuna, drained, flaked
			garlic powder
			oregano
2 oz.	(	57 g)	Gruyère cheese, grated

Will fill a 12" (30 cm) pizza crust.

Sauces, Relishes and Pickles

TOMATO KETCHUP I

Combine in a small saucepan:

| 1 | (| 1) | small onion, finely chopped |
| 6 tbsp. | (| 90 mL) | water |

Cook, stirring occasionally, until tender and all liquid has been absorbed. Transfer to blender; blend until smooth.

Combine in saucepan:

| 2 | (| 2) | medium cooking apples, peeled, cored, sliced |
| 6 tbsp. | (| 90 mL) | unsweetened concentrated apple juice, defrosted |

Cook and stir until apples are soft and juice has been absorbed. Remove from heat. Add:

½ tsp.	(	2 mL)	dry mustard
½ tsp.	(	2 mL)	cinnamon
¼ tsp.	(	1 mL)	allspice
¼ tsp.	(	1 mL)	nutmeg
¼ tsp.	(	1 mL)	salt
			pinch of cloves
			pinch of cayenne

Blend until smooth. Add the onion and:

| 4 tbsp. | (| 60 mL) | vinegar |
| 5½ oz. | (| 156 mL) | tomato paste |

Bring to a boil, then simmer and stir about 5 minutes. Pour into hot clean containers. Cover and cool to room temperature. Refrigerate or freeze. This will keep in refrigerator for at least 2 weeks. Makes two 8-oz. (250 mL) jars.

TOMATO KETCHUP II

Combine in a large stainless steel pot:

10 lbs.	(4.5 kg)	ripe tomatoes, blanched, peeled, cut in pieces
2	(2)	medium onions, peeled, finely chopped
2	(2)	sweet red peppers, seeded, finely chopped

Bring to a boil, then cook over medium heat until tender, stirring often. Press through a sieve.

Add:

⅔ cup	(150 mL)	unsweetened concentrated apple juice, defrosted
1½ cups	(375 mL)	vinegar
1 tsp.	(5 mL)	salt
¼ tsp.	(1 mL)	cayenne

Tie securely in a bag:

2 tsp.	(10 mL)	mixed pickling spice
1½ tsp.	(7 mL)	celery seed
1½ tsp.	(7 mL)	mustard seed
2"	(5 cm)	cinnamon stick

Add to hot mixture. Boil rapidly, stirring often, until thick, 1-1¼ hours. Remove spice bag. Pour into hot clean containers. Cover and cool to room temperature. Refrigerate or freeze. This will keep in refrigerator for at least 2 weeks. Makes about seven 8-oz. (250 mL) jars or bottles.

CHILI SAUCE I

(using fresh tomatoes)

Combine in a large stainless steel pot:

8 lbs.	(	3.5 kg)	ripe tomatoes, blanched, peeled, cut in pieces
2	(	2)	green peppers, seeded, finely chopped
1	(	1)	sweet red pepper, seeded, finely chopped
2	(	2)	large onions, peeled, finely chopped

Bring to a boil, then cook over medium heat until tender, stirring often.

Add:

¾ cup	(	175 mL)	unsweetened concentrated apple juice, defrosted
1⅔ cups	(	400 mL)	vinegar
1 tbsp.	(	15 mL)	dry mustard
1 tsp.	(	5 mL)	cinnamon
1 tsp.	(	5 mL)	allspice
1 tsp.	(	5 mL)	ginger
½ tsp.	(	2 mL)	ground cloves
¼ tsp.	(	1 mL)	cayenne
1 tsp.	(	5 mL)	salt

Cook over medium heat, stirring often, until thick, 1-1¼ hours. Pour into hot clean containers. Cover and cool to room temperature. Refrigerate or freeze. This will keep in refrigerator for at least 2 weeks. Makes about five 16-oz. (500 mL) jars.

CHILI SAUCE II

(using canned tomatoes)

In a stainless steel pot, combine:

28 oz.	(	796 mL)	canned plum tomatoes, drained, crushed
1 cup	(	250 mL)	finely sliced celery
1	(	1)	medium green pepper, seeded, finely chopped
1	(	1)	medium onion, peeled, finely chopped
½ cup	(	125 mL)	vinegar
6 tbsp.	(	90 mL)	unsweetened concentrated apple juice, defrosted
1 tsp.	(	5 mL)	salt
1 tbsp.	(	15 mL)	mixed pickling spices (tied in bag)
¼ tsp.	(	1 mL)	cayenne

Bring to a boil; continue to boil gently until thickened, about 45 minutes, stirring often. Remove spice bag. Pour into hot clean containers. Cover and cool to room temperature. Refrigerate or freeze. This will keep in refrigerator for at least 2 weeks. Makes three 8-oz. (250 mL) jars.

APPLE-CRANBERRY SAUCE

Cook over medium heat for 8 minutes, stirring occasionally:

2	(	2)	medium apples, peeled, cored and finely chopped
1 cup	(	250 mL)	unsweetened concentrated apple juice, defrosted

Add:

2 cups	(	500 mL)	cranberries, fresh OR frozen

Boil gently until the skins of the berries burst and the sauce is thick. Chill before using.

For breakfast, serve with toast or pancakes. For dinner, serve with roast chicken or roast turkey. Makes 2 cups (500 mL).

CRANBERRY JELLY

Combine in a cup:
- 6 tbsp. (90 mL) water
- 1 tbsp. (15 mL) gelatine (1 envelope)

Place in a saucepan:
- 2 cups (500 mL) cranberries, fresh OR frozen
- 1 cup (250 mL) unsweetened concentrated apple juice, defrosted

Boil gently until the skins of the berries burst, about 5 minutes. Add gelatine mixture. Stir until gelatine dissolves. Pour into a mould that has been rinsed in cold water. Chill until set. Makes about 2 cups (500 mL).

CRANBERRY SAUCE

Place in a saucepan:
- 12 oz. (340 g) cranberries, fresh OR frozen
- 1¼ cups (300 mL) unsweetened concentrated apple juice, defrosted

Boil gently until the skins of the berries burst, about 5 minutes. Chill before using. Makes 2½ cups (625 mL).

SPICED CRANBERRY SAUCE

Place in a saucepan:
- 12 oz. (340 g) cranberries, fresh OR frozen
- 1¼ cups (300 mL) unsweetened concentrated apple juice, defrosted

Tie in a cheesecloth bag:
- 2 (2) whole cloves
- 2 (2) whole allspice
- 2" (5 cm) cinnamon stick

Add spices to cranberries. Boil gently until the berries burst, about 5 minutes. Remove spice bag. Chill. Makes 2½ cups (625 mL).

CRANBERRY CHUTNEY

Combine in a saucepan:

12 oz.	(	340 g)	cranberries, fresh OR frozen
1	(	1)	small onion, chopped
⅓ cup	(	75 mL)	coarsely chopped walnuts
½ cup	(	125 mL)	raisins
⅔ cup	(	150 mL)	unsweetened concentrated apple juice, defrosted
2 tbsp.	(	30 mL)	lemon juice
2 tbsp.	(	30 mL)	water
⅛ tsp.	(	0.5 mL)	cloves
			pinch of cayenne

Boil gently until the berries burst and mixture thickens. Ladle into clean jars. Cool to room temperature. Refrigerate or freeze. Will keep in refrigerator for 3 weeks. Makes three 8-oz. (250 jars).

PEACH CHUTNEY

Combine in a deep stainless steel saucepan:

2 lbs.	(	1 kg)	peaches, peeled, pitted, diced
2	(	2)	apples, peeled, cored, diced
1 cup	(	250 mL)	vinegar
½ cup	(	125 mL)	unsweetened concentrated pineapple juice, defrosted
2"	(	5 cm)	cinnamon stick
8	(	8)	whole cloves
2	(	2)	pinches of cayenne

Bring to a boil; boil gently until thick, about 1 hour, stirring frequently. Discard cinnamon stick. Pour into hot clean containers. Cover and cool to room temperature. Refrigerate or freeze. Will keep in refrigerator for 2 weeks. Makes about four 8-oz. (250 mL) jars.

MUSTARD BEAN PICKLES

Remove ends and strings; cut into 1½"(4 cm) lengths:
- **2 lbs.   (1 kg)   wax beans**

Wash; cover with least possible amount of boiling water; cook until just tender, 18-20 minutes. Drain. Mix until smooth:
- **½ cup   (125 mL)   all-purpose flour**
- **⅓ cup   (75 mL)   dry mustard**
- **1 tsp.   (5 mL)   turmeric**
- **1 tsp.   (5 mL)   salt**
- **1½ cups   (375 mL)   unsweetened concentrated apple juice, defrosted**

Bring to a boil:
- **2¼ cups   (550 mL)   vinegar**
- **2 tsp.   (10 mL)   celery seed**

Stir in mustard mixture, cook and stir until thick. Add drained beans; bring to a boil. Pour into hot clean containers. Cover and cool to room temperature. Freeze until needed. Makes about four 16-oz. (500 mL) jars.

GREEN TOMATO PICKLES

Wash and slice thinly:
- **4 lbs.   (1.8 kg)   green tomatoes**
- **2   (2)   large onions, peeled**

Sprinkle with:
- **¼ cup   (60 mL)   salt**

Mix well. Let stand 12 hours or overnight. Drain. Wash with plenty of water. Drain in a colander. Heat to boiling point:
- **2   (2)   green peppers, thinly sliced**
- **3   (3)   sweet red peppers, thinly sliced**
- **1½ cups   (375 ml)   unsweetened concentrated apple juice, defrosted**
- **1½ cups   (375 mL)   vinegar**

TOMATO PICKLES (continued)

Add the tomatoes, onions and:
- 3" (7.6 cm) cinnamon stick
- 1½ tsp. (7 mL) dry mustard

Tie securely in a cheesecloth bag and add to hot tomato mixture:
- 1 tbsp. (15 mL) chopped peeled ginger root
- 1 tbsp. (15 mL) whole cloves
- 1½ tsp. (7 mL) celery seeds

Bring to a boil, then simmer gently for 1 hour, stirring frequently. Pour into hot clean containers. Cover and cool to room temperature. Freeze until needed. Makes eight 8-oz.(250 mL) jars.

BREAD AND BUTTER PICKLES

Wash; cut crosswise into paper-thin slices:
- 12 (12) medium cucumbers, unpeeled
- 4 (4) medium onions, peeled

Add and mix well:
- ¼ cup (60 mL) salt

Refrigerate overnight. Drain vegetables. Rinse in plenty of cold water. Drain again thoroughly.

Combine:
- 1¼ cups (300 mL) vinegar
- 1¼ cups (300 mL) unsweetened concentrated apple juice, defrosted
- 2 tsp. (30 mL) mustard seed
- 1½ tsp. (7 mL) celery seed
- ½ tsp. (2 mL) allspice
- ¼ tsp. (1 mL) cloves

Heat to a boil. Gradually add drained vegetables, keeping just below boiling point. (Otherwise, boiling will soften pickles.) Cook 10 minutes, stirring a little. Place in hot clean containers. Cover and cool to room temperature. Freeze until needed. Makes about four 16-oz. (500 mL) jars.

PICKLED ONIONS

Wash; drain and cover with boiling water:
- **2 qts.** (**2 L**) small white onions

Let stand 5 minutes, drain, cover with cold water and peel. Make a solution of:
- **1 qt.** (**1 L**) of the boiling water
- **½ cup** (**125 mL**) salt

Add onions and let stand 24 hours. Drain. Rinse thoroughly with cold water and drain.

Combine in a stainless steel pot:
- **2 tbsp.** (**30 mL**) mixed pickling spices (tied in bag)
- **3 cups** (**750 mL**) white vinegar
- **⅓ cup** (**75 mL**) unsweetened concentrated pineapple juice, defrosted

Heat spice mixture to boiling, then simmer 1 minute. Remove spices. Add onions and **bring just to boiling point**. Pack onions in hot clean containers and cover with the hot liquid. Cover and cool to room temperature. Freeze until needed. Makes about three to four 16-oz. (500 mL) jars.

QUICK BEET RELISH

Combine in a medium-sized saucepan:
- **2 cups** (**500 mL**) coarsely chopped unsweetened canned OR cooked beets
- **3 tbsp.** (**45 ml**) minced onions
- **3 tbsp.** (**45 mL**) prepared horseradish
- **4 tbsp.** (**60 mL**) vinegar
- **2½ tbsp.** (**38 mL**) unsweetened concentrated apple juice, defrosted
- **½ tsp.** (**2 mL**) dry mustard
- pinch of cayenne

Bring to a boil, reduce to medium-low, cook and stir 5 minutes. Serve hot or cold. Serves 4.

PICKLED BEETS

Cut off the stems within 1" (2.5 cm) of:
- 6 (6) **medium-sized beets**

Scrub them. Pour enough boiling water to cover about ⅔ the depth of beets. Cover and cook until tender, 40-50 minutes. When done, cool beets a little and rub off skins. Slice or dice enough beets to measure 4 cups (1 L). Drop beets into 2 hot clean containers.

Combine in a saucepan; bring to a boil, then gently boil 5 minutes:
- 1 cup (250 mL) **vinegar**
- ½ cup (125 mL) **unsweetened concentrated apple juice, defrosted**
- ½ cup (125 mL) **water**
- ½ tsp (2 mL) **salt**
- 16 (16) **whole cloves (tied in a bag)**

Remove bag. Pour hot liquid over beets. Cover and cool to room temperature. Freeze until needed. Makes two 16-oz. (500 mL) jars.

APPLE-HORSERADISH RELISH

Wash, peel, core and thinly slice:
- 4 (4) **medium cooking apples**

Combine in saucepan with:
- ½ cup (125 mL) **minced celery**
- 2 tbsp. (30 mL) **unsweetened concentrated apple juice, defrosted**
- 2 tbsp. (30 mL) **water**

Bring to a boil; reduce heat to medium-low. Cook and stir until all liquid has evaporated, about 15 minutes. Mash.

Add:
- 3 tbsp. (45 mL) **prepared horseradish**
- 1 tsp. (5 mL) **lemon juice**

Cook and stir 2 minutes. Serve hot or cold. Delicious with pork or beef. Makes 2¼ cups (550 ml).

ZUCCHINI RELISH

Wash, put through the coarsest blade of food grinder or finely chop:

3 lbs.	(1.5 kg)	zucchini
1	(1)	large green pepper, seeded
1½	(1½)	sweet red pepper, seeded
3	(3)	medium onions, peeled

Cover with water and add:

| 3 tbsp. | (45 mL) | salt |

Stir to dissolve salt. Cover and refrigerate overnight. Drain well. Rinse in plenty of water, drain thoroughly. Cover with the least possible amount of boiling water. Cook until just tender, 18-20 minutes. Drain.

Mix until smooth:

| ½ cup | (125 mL) | all-purpose flour |
| ¾ cup | (175 mL) | unsweetened concentrated apple juice, defrosted (1st amount) |

Add:

¾ cup	(175 mL)	unsweetened concentrated apple juice, defrosted (2nd amount)
2¼ cups	(550 mL)	vinegar
1½ tsp.	(7 mL)	celery seed
1½ tsp.	(7 mL)	mustard seed
2	(2)	pinches of cayenne

Cook and stir apple juice mixture until thick. Add drained vegetables. Bring just to boiling point, then simmer 5 minutes. Pour into hot clean containers. Cover and cool to room temperature. Freeze until needed. Makes about four 16-oz. (500 mL) jars.

Jams and Sweet Sauces

RHUBARB-STRAWBERRY JAM

Bring to a boil, reduce heat, cover and simmer 20 minutes:
- 1 lb. (500 g) sliced rhubarb (4 cups [1 L])
- ½ cup (125 mL) unsweetened concentrated apple juice, defrosted

Wash, hull and measure:
- 2 cups (500 mL) sliced strawberries

Crush strawberries with a potato masher. Stir into rhubarb mixture. Cover and cook 5 minutes.

Combine:
- 4 tbsp. (60 mL) unsweetened concentrated apple juice, defrosted
- 1½ tbsp. (22 mL) gelatine

Add gelatine mixture to hot fruit mixture; cook and stir 2 minutes. Ladle into clean 6-oz. jars. Cool to room temperature. Refrigerate or freeze. Will keep in refrigerator for at least 2 weeks. Makes four 6-oz. (175 mL) jars.

See photograph on page 16A.

RHUBARB-PINEAPPLE JAM

From above recipe, omit both amounts of apple juice and strawberries and substitute concentrated pineapple juice and unsweetened crushed pineapple, well-drained.

STRAWBERRY JAM

Combine:
4 tbsp.	(	60 mL)	unsweetened concentrated apple juice, defrosted
1½ tbsp.	(	22 mL)	gelatine

In a saucepan, combine:
1 cup	(	250 mL)	crushed strawberries
1½ cups	(	375 mL)	sliced strawberries
½ cup	(	125 mL)	unsweetened concentrated apple juice, defrosted

Bring to a boil, then simmer and stir 10 minutes. Stir in gelatine mixture; cook and stir 2 minutes. Ladle into clean 6-oz. (175 mL) jars. Cool to room temperature. Refrigerate or freeze. Will keep in refrigerator for at least 2 weeks. Makes about four 6-oz. (175 mL) jars.

PEACH JAM

Wash, blanch 1 minute, drain, peel, pit and slice enough to make:
4.5 lbs.	(	2 kg)	peaches (16-17 medium)

Add:
1¼ cup	(	300 mL)	unsweetened concentrated pineapple juice, defrosted
¼ cup	(	60 mL)	unsweetened concentrated orange juice, defrosted
5 tbsp.	(	75 mL)	lemon juice
2	(	2)	cinnamon sticks, 3½" (9 cm) each

Bring to a rolling boil. Continue to boil on high heat, stirring occasionally, until thick, about 25 to 30 minutes. Discard cinnamon sticks. Pour into hot clean jars to within ¼" (6 mm) from top. Cover and cool to room temperature. Refrigerate or freeze. Will keep in refrigerator for at least 2 weeks. Makes five 8-oz. (250 mL) jars.

See photograph on page 16A.

PLUM JAM

Wash, pit, and cut into quarters:
- **4 cups** (**1 L**) **prune plums**
- **½ cup** (**125 mL**) **unsweetened concentrated apple juice, defrosted**

Bring to a boil and boil until thick, stirring occasionally, about 18 minutes. Pour into hot clean jars to within ¼" (6 mm) of top rim. Cover and cool to room temperature. Refrigerate or freeze. Will keep in refrigerator for at least 2 weeks. Makes about three 8-oz. (250 mL) jars.

See photograph on page 16A.

PEACH SAUCE

Cook, stirring occasionally, until soft:
- **1** (**1**) **large peach, peeled, pitted and sliced**
- **6 tbsp.** (**90 mL**) **unsweetened concentrated pineapple juice, defrosted**
- **⅔ cup** (**150 mL**) **water**

Blend or mash until smooth.

Combine:
- **2 tsp.** (**10 mL**) **cornstarch**
- **1 tbsp.** (**15 mL**) **unsweetened concentrated pineapple juice, defrosted**

Stir cornstarch mixture into peach mixture. Bring to a boil, simmer and stir until thick. Remove from heat.

Add:
- **¼ tsp.** (**1 mL**) **almond extract**

Serve warm or cold. Makes 1 cup (250 mL).

PEAR SAUCE

Cook, stirring occasionally, until soft enough to crush with a fork:
1	(	1)	**medium pear, peeled, cored, sliced**
⅓ cup	(	75 mL)	**unsweetened concentrated apple juice, defrosted**
1 cup	(	250 mL)	**unsweetened pineapple juice**

Turn off heat. Crush with a potato masher or blend until smooth.

Combine until dissolved:
4 tbsp.	(	60 mL)	**unsweetened pineapple juice**
2 tbsp.	(	30 mL)	**cornstarch**

Gradually stir cornstarch mixture into pear mixture. Bring to a boil; reduce heat to medium-low. Cook, stirring a little, for 2 minutes. Makes 1⅔ cups (400 mL).

ORANGE SAUCE

Combine until smooth:
5 tsp.	(	25 mL)	**cornstarch**
½ cup	(	125 mL)	**unsweetened concentrated orange juice, defrosted**

Add:
1 cup	(	250 mL)	**water**
2 tsp.	(	10 mL)	**lemon juice**

Cook and stir until sauce thickens and boils. Boil and stir 1 minute longer.

Peel, separate segments and remove membranes of:
1	(	1)	**orange**

Cut each orange segment into 3 pieces; discard seeds. Add to orange sauce. Makes about 1¾ cups (425 mL).

MAPLE SAUCE

Combine in a small saucepan:
- **3½ tsp.** (**17 mL**) **cornstarch**
- **5 tbsp.** (**75 mL**) **unsweetened concentrated apple juice, defrosted**

Add:
- **1⅓ cups** (**325 mL**) **unsweetened pineapple juice**

Cook and stir cornstarch mixture over medium heat until it thickens and boils. Boil and stir for 1 minute. Remove from heat.

Add:
- **½ tsp.** (**2 mL**) **maple extract**
- **¼ tsp.** (**1 mL**) **vanilla**

Serve hot or cold. Makes about 1¼ cups (300mL).

CHOCOLATE SAUCE

Combine in a small saucepan:
- **3½ tsp.** (**17 mL**) **cornstarch**
- **4 tbsp.** (**60 mL**) **warm water**

Add:
- **3 tbsp.** (**45 mL**) **cocoa**

Gradually stir in until blended:
- **¾ cup** (**175 mL**) **hot water**

Stir in:
- **½ cup** (**125 mL**) **unsweetened concentrated apple juice, defrosted**

Cook and stir chocolate mixture over medium heat until it thickens and boils. Boil and stir 1 minute. Remove from heat; add:
- **½ tsp.** (**2 mL**) **vanilla**

Serve hot or cold. Use on desserts and ice cream. Makes 1⅛ cups (275 mL).

Pastry and Pies

TENDER PIE PASTRY

Sift into a mixing bowl:
- 1 cup (250 mL) all-purpose flour
- ¼ tsp. (1 mL) baking powder

Cut in with a pastry blender until the size of small peas:
- 5 tbsp. (75 mL) butter, margarine OR shortening

Beat together with a fork:
- 1 (1) egg yolk
- 2 tbsp. (30 mL) water

Gradually add to flour mixture as you work quickly with your fingertips, mixing just enough to hold ingredients together. Press into a ball. Wrap in plastic and refrigerate for 30 minutes. Roll dough from centre outwards to ⅛" (3 mm) thick. Fold in half; fit loosely into a 9" (23 cm) pie plate.

For a plain crust, trim off excess pastry. For a fluted crust, roll edge under and on rim of plate. Flute edge by using thumb and index finger of one hand on the outside and index finger of other hand on the inside edge of pastry. Bake according to recipe chosen.

BAKED PIE SHELL

Prick pie shell all over with a fork. Bake at 400°F (200°C) until a light brown, 12-15 minutes.

PEACH PIE

Prepare Baked Pie shell, page 62 or Volume 1, page 6 or 7.

Scald in boiling water for 1 minute, dip in cold water, peel and slice into top of double boiler:
        1 (1) peach

Add:
        ½ cup (125 mL) unsweetened concentrated apple juice, defrosted
        3 tbsp. (45 mL) unsweetened pineapple juice

Over direct heat, bring to a boil, then stir and cook over medium-low heat for 5 minutes. Blend or purée until smooth. Return to double boiler; place over boiling water.

Combine until smooth:
        3 tbsp. (45 mL) cornstarch
        3 tbsp. (45 mL) unsweetened pineapple juice

Stir cornstarch mixture into hot fruit mixture. Cook and stir over boiling water until glaze thickens. Cover and cook 10 minutes. Remove from heat.

Scald, peel and slice each into 8 wedges:
        7-8 (7-8) peaches, depending on size

Arrange peach wedges in an attractive circular pattern in baked pie shell. Spoon half of the glaze over peaches. Repeat with remainder of peaches and glaze. Chill until set.

Serve as is or use a pastry bag fitted with a large fluted tube, pipe decoratively around edge of pie:
        Whipped Cream, prepare half of recipe on page 73, OR
        Mock Whipped Cream, Volume 1, page 30

Serves 6.

FOR AN EVEN CRUMB CRUST

Spread crumb mixture over pie pan. Press another pan (same size) onto the crumb mixture to ensure an even pie crust. Remove the second pan.

STRAWBERRY BAVARIAN PIE

Prepare Baked Pie Shell, page 62 or Crumb Crust, Volume 1, page 8.
Combine:
- 4 tbsp. (60 mL) unsweetened concentrated apple juice, defrosted
- 1 tbsp. (15 mL) gelatine (1 envelope)

With a masher, crush:
- 3 cups (750 mL) fresh strawberries

Heat half of the crushed strawberries until hot; stir in the gelatine mixture; cook and stir 2 minutes. Add to remaining crushed strawberries; mix well; chill until partially set.

Whip until thick and fluffy:
- 1 cup (250 mL) chilled whipping cream

Fold half of whipped cream into partially set mixture. Pour into pie shell. Chill until set. Serve as is or use a pastry bag fitted with a large fluted tube, pipe remaining whipped cream decoratively around edge of pie. Serves 6.

RHUBARB BAVARIAN PIE

Prepare Baked Pie Shell, page 62 or Crumb Crust, Volume 1, page 8.
Bring to a boil, reduce heat, cover and simmer 20 minutes:
- 1 lb. (500 g) rhubarb, sliced 1" (2.5 cm) chunks
- ½ cup (125 mL) unsweetened concentrated apple juice, defrosted

Combine:
- 4 tbsp. (60mL) unsweetened concentrated apple juice, defrosted
- 1 tbsp. (15 mL) gelatine (1 envelope)

Stir gelatine mixture into hot rhubarb mixture. Cook and stir 2 minutes. Chill until partially set.

Pour into a bowl; place in freezer until thoroughly chilled:
- ½ cup (125 mL) evaporated milk, 2% m.f.

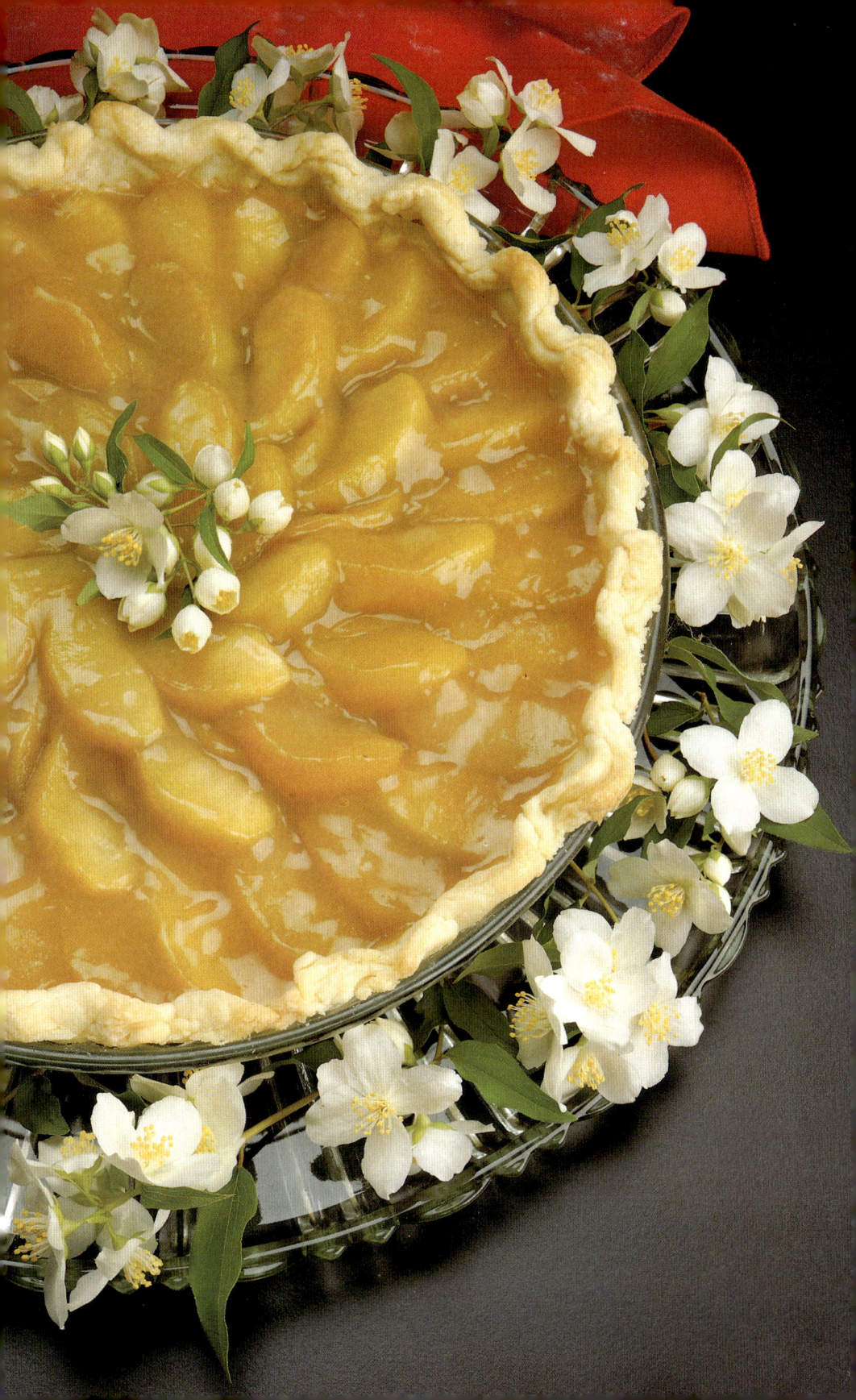

Apple Pie, page 66

RHUBARB BAVARIAN PIE (continued)

Whip until thick and fluffy. Fold into partially set rhubarb mixture. Pour into pie shell or crumb crust. Chill until set.

Serve as is or using a pastry bag fitted with a large fluted tube, pipe decoratively around edge of pie:

    Whipped Cream, prepare half of recipe, page 73 OR
    Mock Whipped Cream, Volume 1, page 30.

Serves 6.

RHUBARB-STRAWBERRY PIE

Prepare Baked Pie Shell, page 62 OR Volume 1, page 6 or 7.

Cover and steam over boiling water, 10 minutes:
    ¾ lb.   (375 g)   **rhubarb, 1" (2.5 cm) chunks**
    ½ cup   (125 mL)   **unsweetened concentrated apple juice, defrosted**

Combine until smooth:
    4 tbsp.   (60 mL)   **unsweetened concentrated apple juice, defrosted**
    3½ tbsp.   (53 mL)   **cornstarch**

Stir cornstarch mixture into the hot rhubarb mixture. Cook and stir gently, 10 minutes.

Wash, hull and measure:
    2 cups   (500 mL)   sliced strawberries

Crush 1 cup (250 mL) of the sliced strawberries. Stir both the crushed and the sliced strawberries into the hot rhubarb mixture. Cover and cook 10 minutes. Cool. Pour into baked pie shell. Chill until set. Garnish with:

    Whipped Cream, prepare half of recipe page 73 OR
    Mock Whipped Cream, Volume 1, page 30.

Serves 6.

BLUEBERRY PIE

Prepare Baked Pie Shell, page 62 OR Volume 1, page 7. Bring to a boil, lower heat to medium-low, cook and stir 3 minutes:
- 1 qt. (1 L) blueberries
- ⅔ cup (150 mL) unsweetened concentrated apple juice, defrosted

Combine until smooth:
- 3 tbsp. (45 mL) cornstarch
- ⅓ cup (75 mL) unsweetened apple juice

Stir cornstarch mixture into hot blueberry mixture. Cook and stir until it thickens and boils. Boil and stir 1 minute. Cool. Pour into pie shell. Chill until firm. Serve as is or garnish with:

Whipped Cream, prepare half of recipe, page 73

Put cream in a pastry bag fitted with a large fluted tube. Pipe cream around edge of pie. Serves 6.

APPLE PIE

Prepare Baked Pie Shell, page 62 OR Volume 1, page 7. Wash, peel, core and slice each into 8 wedges:
- 7 (7) medium apples

Combine in a large saucepan:
- ¾ cup (175 mL) unsweetened concentrated apple juice, defrosted
- ½ cup (125 mL) water

Bring to a boil. Add half the apple wedges. Lower heat to medium. Cook and stir a little, until a fork can penetrate an apple wedge, about 4 minutes. Skim apples out onto a plate. Repeat with remaining apples. To make sauce, combine:
- 2 tbsp. (30 mL) cornstarch
- 4 tbsp. (60 mL) water

Stir cornstarch mixture into hot juice. Cook; stir until thick. Add:
- ½ tsp. (2 mL) vanilla

Remove from heat. Arrange cooked apple wedges in a circular pattern in baked pie shell. Spoon part of the sauce over apples. Repeat until all apples and sauce are used. Chill. Serves 6.

See photograph on page 64A.

SOUR CREAM PINEAPPLE PIE
(using sour cream, 5.5% m.f.)

Prepare Baked Pie Shell, page 62, OR Volume 1, page 6 or 7. Drain well:

| 6 | (| 6) | slices of canned unsweetened pineapple |

Combine in a double boiler:

| 5 tbsp. | (| 75 mL) | all-purpose flour |
| 1 cup | (| 250 mL) | sour cream, 5.5% m.f. |

Beat until smooth. Cook and stir over boiling water until thick. Beat until blended:

| 2 | (| 2) | egg yolks |
| 5 tbsp. | (| 75 mL) | unsweetened concentrated pineapple juice, defrosted |

Add hot sour cream mixture, about 2 tbsp. (30 mL) at a time, mixing well after each addition. Return to double boiler. Cover and cook 4 minutes. Remove from heat. Add:

| ¼ tsp. | (| 1 mL) | almond extract |

Beat until blended. Cool. Place 4 slices of pineapple in baked pie shell. Break up the remaining 2 slices to fill all spaces. Spread cooled filling over pineapple. Top with Pineapple Meringue, recipe follows. Serves 6.

PINEAPPLE MERINGUE

Beat until soft peaks form:

| 2 | (| 2) | egg whites |

Add and beat until stiff:

| ½ tsp. | (| 2 mL) | cornstarch |
| ¼ tsp. | (| 1 mL) | cream of tartar |

Beat in:

| 2 tbsp. | (| 30 mL) | unsweetened concentrated pineapple juice, defrosted |

Spread meringue* over pie filling. Broil about 8" (20 cm) from heat until nicely browned, about 3-4 minutes.

* Make sure that meringue is sealed to entire circumference of pie shell, otherwise it will shrink away from shell during baking or broiling.

LEMON PIE

Prepare Baked Pie Shell, page 62, OR Crumb Crust, Volume 1, page 8.

In top of double boiler, combine:

1 cup	(	250 mL)	unsweetened pineapple juice
⅔ cup	(	150 mL)	unsweetened concentrated apple juice, defrosted
4 tbsp.	(	60 mL)	lemon juice
1 tbsp.	(	15 mL)	grated lemon rind

Place over direct heat until hot, then over boiling water.

Combine until smooth:

| 5 tbsp. | (| 75 mL) | cornstarch |
| 6 tbsp. | (| 90 mL) | unsweetened concentrated apple juice, defrosted |

Stir cornstarch mixture into hot juice. Cook and stir over boiling water until thick. Cover and cook 10 minutes. Beat:

    2 (2) egg yolks

Add a little hot juice mixture to yolks; mix; return to hot juice mixture. Cook and stir 2 minutes. Remove from heat. Cool before pouring into chilled pie shell. Cover with Lemon Meringue, recipe follows.

Serves 6.

LEMON MERINGUE

Beat until stiff:

2	(	2)	egg whites
½ tsp.	(	2 mL)	grated lemon rind
¼ tsp.	(	1 mL)	cream of tartar
½ tsp.	(	2 mL)	cornstarch

Gradually beat in:

    2 tbsp. (30 mL) unsweetened concentrated apple juice, defrosted

Swirl meringue decoratively over filling, touching all edges of pie crust. Bake at 350°F (180°C) until a delicate brown, about 10-15 minutes.

RAISIN MERINGUE PIE

Prepare Baked Pie Shell, page 62 OR Volume I, page 6 or 7.

Bring to a boil; reduce to medium-low:
- 1 cup (250 mL) raisins
- 4 tbsp. (60 mL) unsweetened concentrated orange juice, defrosted
- ½ cup (125 mL) water
- ¼ tsp. (1 mL) grated orange rind

Combine:
- 1 tbsp. (15 mL) cornstarch
- 4 tbsp. (60 mL) water

Stir cornstarch mixture into raisin mixture. Cook and stir until it thickens and boils.

Beat:
- 2 (2) egg yolks

Add about 2 tbsp. (30 mL) hot liquid to egg yolks. Mix until blended; stir back into hot mixture. Cook and stir 3 minutes. Cool to lukewarm. Pour into baked pie shell. Cover with Nut Meringue, recipe follows. Serves 6.

NUT MERINGUE

Beat until soft peaks form:
- 2 (2) egg whites

Add and beat until stiff:
- ½ tsp. (2 mL) cornstarch
- ¼ tsp. (1 mL) cream of tartar

Beat in:
- 2 tbsp. (30 mL) unsweetened concentrated orange juice, defrosted

Fold in:
- ¼ cup (60 mL) finely chopped pecans OR walnuts

Spread meringue over raisin filling, touching all edges of the crust. Broil about 8" (20 cm) from heat until browned, 3-4 minutes.

PUMPKIN CHIFFON PIE

Prepare Baked Pie Shell, page 62, OR Volume 1, page 6 or 7.

Combine in a cup:

| ¼ cup | (| 60 mL) | unsweetened concentrated apple juice, defrosted |
| 1 tbsp. | (| 15 mL) | gelatine (1 envelope) |

In top of double boiler, beat well with a wire whip:

| 2 | (| 2) | large eggs |

Add and beat until blended:

1½ cups	(	375 mL)	mashed, cooked OR canned pumpkin
½ cup	(	125 mL)	unsweetened concentrated apple juice, defrosted
½ tsp.	(	2 mL)	cinnamon
¼ tsp.	(	1 mL)	nutmeg
¼ tsp.	(	1 mL)	ginger
2	(	2)	pinches of cloves

Cook and stir over boiling water until smooth and thick. Add gelatin mixture, stirring until completely dissolved. Chill until thick but not stiff.

Add to pumpkin mixture and beat on high speed until volume doubles:

| ½ cup | (| 125 mL) | instant skim milk powder |

Pour pumpkin filling into pie shell. Chill until firm. Garnish with:

Whipped Cream, prepare half of recipe page 73 OR Mock Whipped Cream, Volume 1, page 30.

Serves 6.

TO COOK PUMPKIN

Wash pumpkin; cut into quarters; remove seeds and fibres. Steam over boiling water until tender, 25-30 minutes. To bake pumpkin place pumpkin quarters, shell side up, in a baking dish. Cover and bake at 325°F (160°C) until tender, about 50 minutes. With either method, when tender, scrape pulp from shell and mash or blend it in a blender.

Puddings and Cheesecakes

STRAWBERRY TRIFLE

Use leftover plain or sponge cake or prepare Plain Cake, page 83 but line the bottom of an 11"x7" (28x18 cm) pan with waxed paper. Bake 25-30 minutes at 350°F (180°C). Turn pan upside down to cool. Remove cake from pan, discard waxed paper.

Wash, pat dry and hull; reserve 12 for topping:
    1 qt. (1 L) **fresh strawberries**

Spread cake with:
    Strawberry Jam, page 58

Cut cake into cubes about ¾" (1.9 cm) and place in a 2-quart. (2 L) serving bowl or return cake (uncut) to baking pan.

Sprinkle top of cake with mixture of:
    6 tbsp. (90 mL) **unsweetened concentrated apple juice, defrosted**
    1 tsp. (5 mL) **cherry extract**
    1 tsp. (5 mL) **brandy extract**

Cover generously with sliced strawberries. Spread Custard Cream, page 73, over berries; cover with plastic wrap; chill 2 hours. To serve, spoon or cut into individual portions; garnish with:
    whipped cream, page 73
    reserved strawberries

Serves 10-12.

PINEAPPLE TRIFLE

Use leftover plain or sponge cake or prepare Plain Cake page 83 but line the bottom of an 11"x7" (28x18 cm) pan with waxed paper. Bake 25-30 minutes at 350°F (180°C). Turn pan upside down to cool. Remove cake from pan; discard waxed paper.

Drain well; reserve juice to make Pineapple Jelly, recipe follows:

19 oz. (540 mL) can unsweetened pineapple slices, chunks OR crushed

For crushed pineapple, pour into a sieve; press pineapple with spoon to release more juice.

Cut cake into cubes about ¾" (1.9 cm) and place in a 2-quart (2 L) serving bowl or return cake (uncut) to baking pan.

Sprinkle top of cake with mixture of:

6 tbsp. (90 mL) unsweetened concentrated pineapple juice, defrosted
1 tsp. (5 mL) cherry extract
1 tsp. (5 mL) brandy extract

Cover with drained pineapple. Pour in Pineapple Jelly mixture, recipe follows; chill until set. Spread Custard Cream, page 73, over jelly; cover with plastic wrap; chill 2 hours. To serve, spoon or cut into individual portions; garnish with:

Whipped Cream, page 73.

Serves 10-12.

PINEAPPLE JELLY

Combine to soften:

6 tbsp. (90 mL) unsweetened concentrated pineapple juice, defrosted
1 tbsp. (15 mL) gelatine (1 envelope)

Measure reserved pineapple juice and add:

boiling water to make 1⅔ cups (400 mL)

Stir hot juice mixture into softened gelatine until gelatine dissolves completely. Pour this pineapple jelly mixture over cake; chill until set.

CUSTARD CREAM

Combine in saucepan until smooth:
- **3 tbsp.** (**45 mL**) cornstarch
- **½ cup** (**125 mL**) milk

Add:
- **1 cup** (**250 mL**) milk

Cook and stir over medium heat until it thickens and boils. Boil and stir 1 minute.

Beat together:
- **2** (**2**) eggs, beaten
- **5 tbsp.** (**75 mL**) unsweetened concentrated pineapple OR apple juice, defrosted

Stir egg mixture into hot milk mixture. Cook and stir for 3 minutes. Remove from heat.

Add:
- **1 tsp.** (**5 mL**) vanilla

Cover to prevent crusting; cool. (To cool quickly place in freezer.) When cooled, fold in:
- **½ cup** (**125 mL**) Whipped Cream, recipe follows

WHIPPED CREAM

Whip until stiff:
- **1 cup** (**250 mL**) whipping cream

Add:
- **1 tsp.** (**5 mL**) unsweetened concentrated pineapple OR apple juice, defrosted

Whip until blended.

CREAMY RICE PUDDING

Combine in a saucepan:
- 4 tbsp. (60 mL) raw long-grain rice, washed
- 4 cups (1 L) milk

Bring to a boil; reduce to medium heat; cook 20 minutes, stirring often. Reduce to low; cook 10 minutes longer. Mix in:
- ½ cup (125 mL) raisins
- ½ tsp. (2 mL) cinnamon

Beat well:
- 2 (2) eggs

Beat in:
- ⅔ cup (150 mL) unsweetened concentrated apple juice, defrosted to room temperature

Stir egg mixture into hot rice mixture. Cook and stir for 3 minutes. Remove from heat, add:
- 1 tsp. (5 mL) vanilla

Serve warm or cold with milk or pouring cream. Serves 6.

STEAMED RHUBARB

Combine in top of double boiler:
- 1 lb. (500 g) rhubarb, in 1" (2.5 cm) lengths
- ½ cup (125 mL) unsweetened concentrated apple juice, defrosted

Cover and steam rhubarb mixture over boiling water for 10 minutes. Mix until smooth:
- 2½ tbsp. (38 ml) cornstarch
- 4 tbsp. (60 mL) unsweetened concentrated apple juice, defrosted

Stir cornstarch mixture into hot rhubarb mixture. Cook and stir until mixture is clear and thick, about 10 minutes. Cover and cook about 5 minutes longer. Cool. Serve as is or with:

Whipped Cream, page 73 OR
Ice Cream, Volume 1, page 57

Serves 3-4.

LEMON SNOW

Combine and stir until completely dissolved:
- 1 tbsp. (15 mL) gelatine (1 envelope)
- 1 cup (250 mL) hot water

Add:
- ½ tsp. (2 mL) grated lemon rind
- 6 tbsp. (90 mL) lemon juice
- ¾ cup (175 mL) unsweetened concentrated pineapple OR apple juice, defrosted

Chill until partially set. Add:
- ⅔ cup (150 mL) instant skim milk powder

Beat until firm peaks form. Pour into a mould. Chill until set, 1 hour. Serves 4-6.

LEMON PUDDING

This pudding separates into 2 layers. There is a layer of lemon custard at the bottom and a layer of cake on top.

Combine:
- 3½ tbsp. (53 mL) all-purpose flour
- ¾ cup (175 mL) unsweetened concentrated apple juice, room temperature
- 1 (1) lemon, grated rind of

Preheat oven to 325°F (160°C).

Beat until stiff:
- 3 (3) egg whites

Beat well:
- 3 (3) egg yolks

Add flour mixture to egg yolks; beat until blended. Gradually stir in:
- 1 cup (250 mL) milk

Fold in stiffly-beaten egg whites. Pour into six custard cups or a 2-quart (2 L) baking dish; place in a pan of hot water; bake until brown, 45-55 minutes. Serves 6.

PUMPKIN PUDDING

This pudding separates into two parts — the cake on the outside encases the pumpkin mixture inside.

Oil bottom of a 1½ quart (1.5 L) baking dish.

Sift together:

1 cup	(250 mL)	all-purpose flour
1 tsp.	(5 mL)	baking powder
¼ tsp.	(1 mL)	baking soda
½ tsp.	(2 mL)	cinnamon
¼ tsp.	(1 mL)	nutmeg
¼ tsp.	(1 mL)	ginger
2	(2)	pinches of cloves

Preheat oven to 350°F (180°C).

Beat until blended:

2	(2)	eggs, beaten
3 tbsp.	(45 mL)	melted butter, margarine OR vegetable oil
1 cup	(250 mL)	unsweetened concentrated apple juice, defrosted to room temperature
2 cups	(500 mL)	mashed, cooked OR canned pumpkin
⅓ cup	(75 mL)	milk

Fold in flour mixture until well blended. Pour into prepared dish. Bake until brown and firm in centre, about 1¼ hours. Serve warm with:

Whipped Cream, page 73.

Serves 6.

CARROT PUDDING

From above recipe, omit nutmeg, ginger, cloves and mashed cooked pumpkin. Beat in with egg mixture:

2 cups	(500 mL)	**mashed cooked carrots**

SELF-SAUCING ORANGE PUDDING

This pudding rises to the top and the sauce settles to the bottom of the dish.

Oil a 2-quart (2 L) pudding or baking dish. Preheat oven to 350°F (180°C). Sift together:
- 1¼ cups (300 mL) all-purpose flour
- 2 tsp. (10 mL) baking powder
- ½ tsp. (2 mL) baking soda

Add:
- ¾ cup (175 mL) raisins

Beat well:
- 1 (1) egg

Beat into egg:
- 3 tbsp. (45 mL) melted butter, margarine OR oil
- 2 tsp. (10 mL) grated orange rind

Add the flour mixture to the egg mixture in two parts, alternating each part with about half of:
- ¾ cup (175 mL) unsweetened concentrated orange juice, room temperature

Fold in until blended after each addition. Pour into prepared pudding or baking dish.

Sprinkle evenly over top of batter:
- 1 tbsp. (15 mL) all-purpose flour

Heat to boiling point:
- ¾ cup (175 mL) unsweetened concentrated orange juice, defrosted
- 1⅓ cups (325 mL) water
- 1 tsp. (5 mL) grated orange rind

Gradually pour orange juice mixture over top of batter. DO NOT STIR! Bake until nicely browned, 45-50 minutes. Serve hot. Serves 6.

SELF-SAUCING LEMON PUDDING

From above recipe, omit orange rind and juice and replace with the same amount of lemon rind and pineapple or apple juice.

NO-BAKE FRUIT CHEESECAKE

Prepare crumb crust, Volume 1, page 8. Pat crumb mixture over bottom and sides of a 9" (23 cm) springform pan. Bake 10 minutes at 350°F (180°C). Chill.

Combine:
- 2 tbsp.   (30 mL)   gelatine (2 envelopes)
- ½ cup   (125 mL) unsweetened concentrated apple juice, defrosted to room temperature

Warm over low heat until gelatine dissolves. Mix in:
- 1 cup   (250 mL) unsweetened pineapple juice

Chill until thick, but not set. Add:
- ⅔ cup   (150 mL) instant skim milk powder

Beat until volume doubles. Chill.

Beat in a double boiler until blended:
- 3   (3)   eggs

Beat in:
- ½ cup   (125 mL) unsweetened concentrated apple juice, defrosted to room temperature
- ¼ cup   (60 mL)   unsweetened pineapple juice
- 1 tsp.   (5 mL)   grated lemon rind

Cook and stir over boiling water until thick. Cool. Using a blender, blend until smooth, the cooled egg mixture and:
- 2¼ cups (500 g)   cottage cheese, 1 % m.f.

Into cottage cheese mixture, fold in the gelatine mixture and:
- ¾ cup   (175 mL) fruit *   1st amount

Pour into baked crumb crust. Cover top with:
- ¾ cup   (175 mL) fruit *   2nd amount

Chill until set before serving, about 2 hours.

Serves 10.

* Fresh sliced peaches, nectarines, apricots, canned unsweetened pineapple chunks, blueberries, etc.

LEMON CHEESECAKE

Prepare Crumb Crust, Volume 1, page 8. Reserve ¼ cup (60 mL) of crumb mixture to sprinkle on top; pat remainder on bottom and sides of a 9" (23 cm) springform pan. Chill.

Preheat oven to 350°F (180°C).

Beat at low speed until smooth:

3x8-oz	(3x250 g)	pkgs. cream cheese, room temperature
4	(4)	egg yolks
1 tbsp.	(15 mL)	grated lemon rind
⅞ cup	(205 mL)	unsweetened concentrated apple juice, room temperature
3 tbsp.	(45 mL)	all-purpose flour

Beat until stiff, about 3 minutes:

4	(4)	egg whites

Fold egg whites into cheese mixture. Pour into prepared crust; sprinkle reserved crumbs over the filling. Bake until centre is firm, about 1 hour. Turn off heat. Leave the cheesecake to cool in the oven for 1 hour with oven door open. Refrigerate 1 hour before serving. Serves 10.

ADJUSTING OVEN SHELVES

For baking cakes and cookies, adjust the oven shelf to as near the middle of the oven as possible before turning on the oven. For baking meringues, adjust the shelf as low as possible.

PREPARING INGREDIENTS

Have all ingredients (measured) at room temperature. For eggs, if necessary to bring to correct temperature, soak eggs in warm water. For milk or juice heat on low until warm.

Cakes

BLACK FOREST CAKE

Oil and lightly flour three 7" or 8" (17 or 20 cm) round cake pans.

Sift together:
1 cup	(	250 mL)	sifted all-purpose flour
⅓ cup	(	75 mL)	cocoa
2½ tsp.	(	12 mL)	baking powder
½ tsp.	(	2 mL)	baking soda

Preheat oven to 350°F (180°C).

Cream until soft and creamy:
    5 tbsp. (75 mL) butter OR margarine

Beat in thoroughly 1 at a time:
    4 (4) large egg yolks

To egg mixture, add the flour mixture in two parts, alternating each part with about half of:
    ⅞ cup (205 mL) unsweetened concentrated apple juice, defrosted to room temperature

Fold in until blended after each addition.

Beat on high speed until frothy, about 30 seconds:
    4 (4) large egg whites

Add and beat until stiff, 2½ minutes:
    ¼ tsp. (1 mL) cream of tartar

Fold into batter quickly and gently. Divide evenly among the 3 pans. Bake until done, 25-30 minutes. Cool 5 minutes; remove cakes from pans; cool. While cakes are cooling prepare cherries.

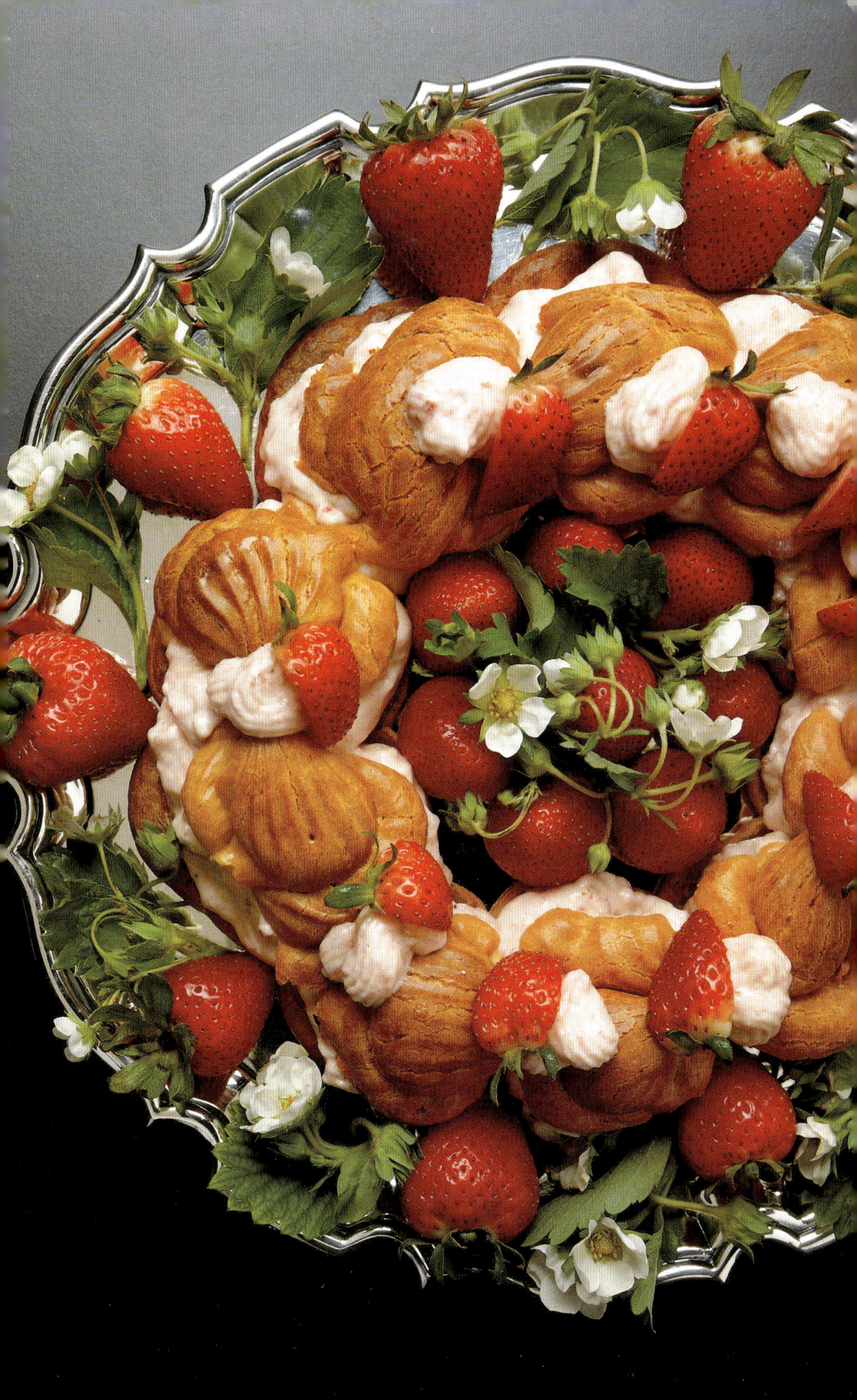

Strawberry Puff Ring, page 92

BLACK FOREST CAKE (continued)

Drain well; remove stones with a cherry pitter from:

   2x14-oz. (2x398 mL)   cans unsweetened Bing cherries
                                      OR 2x10-oz. (2x300 g) frozen unsweetened pitted cherries, defrosted and drained
                                      OR 1¼ lbs. (625 g) fresh Bing cherries, pitted

Reserve 12 cherries to decorate top. Cut remainder into halves.

Sprinkle each layer of cake with:

   2 tbsp. (30 mL)   kirsch OR about 2 tbsp. (30 mL) of a mixture of 6 tbsp. (90 mL) unsweetened concentrated pineapple juice, defrosted and 1 tsp. (5 mL) cherry extract, 1 tsp. (5 mL) brandy flavour

Whip until stiff:

   1¾ cups (425 mL)   whipping cream

Place 1 layer of cake on a serving plate; spread it with ¼ of the whipped cream; cover with ½ of the cherries. Repeat with second layer of cake. Cover with third layer. Frost top and sides with ½ of remaining whipped cream. Put the rest in a pastry bag fitted with a fluted tube. Pipe 12 rosettes around the edge of the cake. Top each rosette with a cherry. Heap carob curls, recipe follows, in the centre. Gently press pieces of carob onto the sides of the cake. Refrigerate. Serves 12.

See photograph on front cover.

CAROB CURLS

In a small container over low heat, melt:

        1 oz. (30 g)   unsweetened plain carob bar

Add and mix well:

        1 tsp. (5 mL)   butter OR margarine

Remove from heat. Allow to cool until firm enough to form into a ¾"x½" (1.9x1.3 cm) deep bar. Place on a flat surface or on a plastic chopping board. Refrigerate until set. Slice carob bar surface with a potato peeler; shave carob into curls. Lift carefully with a toothpick or a knife blade. Arrange decoratively on cake.

MARBLE CAKE

Oil and lightly flour a 9" (23 cm) tube pan.

Sift together:
- 1¾ cups (425 mL) sifted all-purpose flour
- 3 tsp. (15 mL) baking powder
- ½ tsp. (2 mL) baking soda

Preheat oven to 350°F (180°C).

Cream until soft and creamy:
- ½ cup (125 mL) **butter OR margarine**

Beat in 1 at a time:
- 4 (4) **egg yolks**

Combine:
- 1 cup (250 mL) **unsweetened concentrated apple juice, room temperature**
- 1 tsp. (5 mL) **vanilla**

Add juice mixture to creamed egg mixture alternating with flour mixture, in two parts, folding after each addition until blended. To ½ of the batter add:
- 1 oz. (28 g) **unsweetened chocolate, melted**

Beat on high speed until frothy, about 30 seconds:
- 4 (4) **egg whites**

Add and beat until stiff, about 2½ minutes:
- ¼ tsp. (1 mL) **cream of tartar**

Fold ½ of the egg white mixture into the light batter and ½ into the dark batter. Place large spoonfuls of each batter into prepared pan, alternating light and dark mixtures. Swirl the back of a spoon through the batter to create a marbled effect. Bake 55-60 minutes. Invert on wire rack for 15 minutes. Remove cake from pan. Frost when cooled with:

Seven Minute Frosting, Volume 1, page 34.

For a marble appearance, melt over low heat:
- 1 oz. (30 g) **unsweetened chocolate**

Pour or drizzle over frosting. Serves 8-10.

PLAIN CAKE

Line bottom of an 8" (20 cm) square or round cake pan with ungreased waxed paper.

Sift into a mixing bowl:
- 1 cup (250 mL) all-purpose flour
- 2 tsp. (10 mL) baking powder
- ¼ tsp. (1 mL) baking soda

Preheat oven to 350°F (180°C).

With a wooden spoon, beat together until blended:
- 3 (3) egg yolks
- 3 tbsp. (45 mL) vegetable oil
- ½ cup (125 mL) unsweetened concentrated apple juice, defrosted to room temperature
- 1 tsp. (5 mL) vanilla

Add to flour mixture; stir until smooth.

Beat on high until frothy, about 30 seconds:
- 3 (3) egg whites

Add and beat until stiff, about 2 minutes:
- ¼ tsp. (1 mL) cream of tartar

Fold egg whites into batter gently and thoroughly. Pour into prepared pan. Gently cut batter with spatula to release large air bubbles. Bake until nicely browned, 35-40 minutes. Turn pan upside down on wire rack to cool, about 50 minutes. Frost as desired. Serves 9.

REMOVING CAKE FROM PAN

To remove cake from pan, place wire rack on the pan. Hold the rack and pan with cloth and turn the two together.

POPPY SEED TORTE

Oil and lightly flour two 8" (20 cm) round cake pans.

Soak 2 hours:
    ⅔ cup   (150 mL)   poppy seeds
    1 cup   (250 mL)   unsweetened concentrated apple juice, defrosted

Sift together:
    1¾ cups   (425 mL)   sifted all-purpose flour
    2¾ tsp.   (14 mL)   baking powder
    ½ tsp.   (2 mL)   baking soda

Preheat oven to 350°F (180°C).

Cream until soft and creamy:
    ½ cup   (125 mL)   butter OR margarine

Add the poppy seed mixture and:
    1 tsp.   (5 mL)   vanilla

Beat until well-blended. Stir in the sifted ingredients.

Beat on high speed until stiff, about 3 minutes:
    4   (4)   large egg whites

Fold egg whites into batter. Pour batter into prepared pans. Bake until done, about 25 minutes. Cool. Spread Custard Cream Filling, recipe follows, between layers. Cover top and sides with Chocolate Whipped Cream, page 85, and toasted sliced almonds, page 85. Serves 8-10.

CUSTARD CREAM FILLING

Pour into top of double boiler:
    ¾ cup   (175 mL)   milk

Place over direct heat until hot, then over boiling water.

Combine until smooth:
    2 tbsp.   (30 mL)   cornstarch
    3 tbsp.   (45 mL)   milk

Stir cornstarch mixture into hot milk. Cook and stir over boiling water until thick. Cover and cook 10 minutes.

CUSTARD CREAM FILLING (continued)

Beat until blended:
- 3-4 (3-4) egg yolks
- 3½ tbsp. (53 mL) unsweetened concentrated apple juice, defrosted

To egg mixture add 2 tbsp. (30 mL) hot mixture; mix well; return to double boiler. Cook and stir 3 minutes. Remove from heat.

Stir in:
- 1 tsp. (5 mL) vanilla

Cool before using to spread between cake layers.

CHOCOLATE WHIPPED CREAM

Beat until stiff:
- 1 cup (250 mL) whipping cream

Warm over low heat until melted:
- 1 oz. (30 g) unsweetened chocolate
- 4 tbsp. (60 mL) unsweetened concentrated apple juice, defrosted

Stir over low heat until well blended. Remove from heat. Mix in 1 tbsp. (15 mL) of the whipped cream. Refrigerate. When chocolate mixture has cooled, fold into the whipped cream.

TOASTED ALMONDS

Spread sliced almonds on a baking sheet in a 350°F (180°C) oven for 8-10 minutes. Stir once or twice for even toasting.

TO CHECK CAKE FOR DONENESS

Insert a toothpick in the centre of the cake at the end of given baking time. If it comes out clean (no batter clinging to it) the cake is done.

ORANGE CAKE

Oil and lightly flour two 8" (20 cm) round cake pans.

Sift together:
- 1⅓ cups (325 mL) all-purpose flour
- 2½ tsp. (12 mL) baking powder
- ½ tsp. (2 mL) baking soda

Preheat oven to 350°F (180°C).

Cream until soft and creamy:
- 6 tbsp. (90 mL) butter OR margarine
- 1 (1) orange, grated rind of

Beat in 1 at a time:
- 2 (2) large egg yolks

Combine:
- ¾ cup (175 mL) unsweetened concentrated orange juice, defrosted to room temperature
- 1 tsp. (5 mL) vanilla

Add juice mixture to creamed yolk mixture alternating with flour mixture, in 2 parts, folding after each addition until blended.

Beat on high speed until frothy, about 30 seconds:
- 4 (4) large egg whites

Add and beat until stiff, about 2½ minutes:
- ¼ tsp. (1 mL) cream of tartar

Fold egg whites into batter. Pour batter into prepared pans. Bake until nicely browned, about 30 minutes. Cool 5 minutes on wire racks. Remove cake from pans. When cool, spread ⅓ of Orange Filling and Topping, page 87, on bottom layer of cake; add top layer; spread remainder on top and sides. Serves 8.

TO FREEZE CAKE

Return cooled cake to the pan in which it was baked; freeze it; remove it from the pan. Wrap cake in a freezer bag or foil and freeze.

ORANGE FILLING AND TOPPING

Combine in a double boiler:
- ¾ cup+1 tbsp. (190 mL) unsweetened concentrated orange juice, defrosted
- 2 tbsp. (30 mL) lemon juice
- ½ tsp. (2 mL) grated orange rind

Place over direct heat until hot, then over boiling water.

Combine in a cup until smooth:
- 2 tbsp. (30 mL) cornstarch
- 6 tbsp. (90 mL) water

Add cornstarch mixture to hot juice mixture. Cook and stir over boiling water until filling thickens and boils. Cover and cook about 10 minutes.

Beat:
- 2 (2) egg yolks

To egg yolks, add about half the hot juice mixture, blend well; return to hot mixture. Cook, stirring gently, 2 minutes. Cool. To cool quickly set pan in ice water.

Beat until stiff:
- ¾ cup (175 mL) whipping cream

Beat the cooled filling mixture until smooth. Fold into the whipped cream. Use ⅓ of filling between layers of cake and the remainder for top and sides.

BAKING HINT

Do not open oven door during first 15 minutes of baking, unless it is for cookies. For small cookies, the oven may be opened after 5 minutes of baking.

LEMON CHIFFON CAKE

Sift before measuring:
    1½ cups (375 mL) all-purpose flour

Add and sift into a large mixing bowl:
    3 tsp. (15 mL) baking powder
    ½ tsp. (2 mL) baking soda

Beat until blended:
    6 (6) large egg yolks
    1 tbsp. (15 mL) grated lemon rind
    ⅓ cup (75 mL) vegetable oil
    1 tsp. (5 mL) vanilla
    ⅞ cup (205 mL) **unsweetened concentrated apple juice, defrosted to room temperature**

Add egg mixture to sifted ingredients. Stir with a wooden spoon to mix, then beat until smooth.

Preheat oven to 325°F (160°C).

Beat on high speed until frothy, about 1 minute:
    8 (8) **large egg whites**

Add and beat until stiff, about 5 minutes:
    ½ tsp. (2 mL) cream of tartar

Fold egg whites into batter quickly and gently. Pour batter into an ungreased 10" (25 cm) tube pan with removable bottom. Gently cut through batter with spatula to release large air bubbles. Bake at 325°F (160°C) for 50 minutes; increase to 350°F (180°C) for 10-13 minutes. Turn pan upside down, placing the tube over a funnel until cool, 1-1½ hours. Use a serrated knife to cut cake. Serves 12-16.

ORANGE CHIFFON CAKE

To make Orange Chiffon Cake, omit lemon rind and apple juice. Substitute grated rind of one orange and same amount of concentrated orange juice.

POPPY SEED CHIFFON CAKE

Soak for 2 hours:
- ½ cup   (125 mL)   poppy seeds
- 1 cup   (250 mL)   unsweetened concentrated apple juice, defrosted

Sift before measuring:
- 1¾ cups   (425 mL)   all-purpose flour

Add to flour and sift into a large mixing bowl:
- 3 tsp.   (15 mL)   baking powder
- ½ tsp.   (2 mL)   baking soda

Make a well in centre of the flour mixture and add the poppy seed mixture and:
- 7   (7)   large egg yolks
- ⅓ cup   (75 mL)   vegetable oil
- 1 tsp.   (5 mL)   vanilla

Stir with a wooden spoon to mix, then beat manually until smooth.

Preheat oven to 325°F (160°C).

Beat on high speed until frothy, about 1 minute:
- 7   (7)   large egg whites

Add and beat until stiff, about 4 minutes:
- ½ tsp.   (2 mL)   cream of tartar

Fold egg whites into batter quickly and gently. Pour batter into an ungreased 10" (25 cm) tube pan with removable bottom. Gently cut through batter with spatula to release large air bubbles. Bake at 325°F (160°C) for 55 minutes; increase to 350°F (180°C) for 10-13 minutes. Turn pan upside down, placing the tube over a funnel until cool, 1-1½ hours. Use a serrated knife to cut cake. Serves 12-16.

TO SEPARATE EGG WHITES AND YOLKS EASILY

Crack the shell and gently drop the egg into a tablespoon, resting over a small dish. Lift the tablespoon gently; the egg white will slide off into the dish leaving the yolk on the tablespoon.

MAPLE WALNUT CHIFFON CAKE

Sift before measuring:
    1½ cups   (375 mL)   all-purpose flour

Add and sift into a large mixing bowl:
    3 tsp.   (15 mL)   baking powder
    ½ tsp.   (2 mL)   baking soda

Mix in:
    ¾ cup   (175 mL)   finely chopped walnuts

Beat together:
    6   (6)   large egg yolks
    ⅓ cup   (75 mL)   vegetable oil
    ¾ cup+1 tbsp.(190 mL)   unsweetened concentrated apple juice, room temperature
    4 tsp.   (20 mL)   maple flavour

Add egg mixture to flour mixture. Stir with a wooden spoon to mix, then beat until blended.

Preheat oven to 325°F (160°C). Beat on high speed until frothy, about 1 minute:
    8   (8)   large egg whites

Add and beat until stiff, about 5 minutes:
    ½ tsp.   (2 mL)   cream of tartar

Fold egg whites into batter quickly and gently. Pour batter into an ungreased 10" (25 cm) tube pan with removable bottom. Gently cut through batter with spatula to release large air bubbles. Bake at 325°F (160°C) for 50 minutes; increase to 350°F (180°C) for 10-13 minutes. Turn pan upside down, placing the tube over a funnel until cool, 1-1½ hours. Use a serrated knife to cut cake. Serves 12-16.

VANILLA CHIFFON CAKE

From above recipe, omit walnuts and maple flavouring. Substitute 2 tsp. (10 mL) of vanilla for the maple flavour.

CHOCOLATE CHIFFON CAKE

Cook and stir until all liquid is absorbed; purée in a blender until mixture is smooth and thick:

| 12 | (12) | pitted dates, finely sliced |
| ½ cup | (125 mL) | unsweetened concentrated apple juice, defrosted |

Combine and sift into a large mixing bowl:

1⅓ cups	(325 mL)	sifted all-purpose flour
7 tbsp.	(105 mL)	cocoa
3 tsp.	(15 mL)	baking powder
¾ tsp.	(4 mL)	baking soda

To the blended date mixture, add:

6	(6)	large egg yolks
⅓ cup	(75 mL)	vegetable oil
⅔ cup	(150 mL)	unsweetened concentrated apple juice, room temperature
1 tsp.	(5 mL)	vanilla

Beat until smooth. Add egg mixture to flour mixture. Stir with a wooden spoon to mix, then beat manually until smooth.

Preheat oven to 325°F (160°C).

Beat on high speed until frothy, about 1 minute:

| 8 | (8) | large egg whites |

Add and beat until stiff, about 5 minutes:

| ½ tsp. | (2 mL) | cream of tartar |

Fold egg whites into batter quickly and gently. Pour into an ungreased 10" (25 cm) tube pan which has a removable bottom. Gently cut through batter with spatula to release large air bubbles. Bake at 325°F (160°C) for 55 minutes; increase to 350°F (180°C) for 10-13 minutes. Turn pan upside down, placing the tube over a funnel until cool, 1-1½ hours. Use a serrated knife to cut cake.

Serves 12-16.

MOCHA CHIFFON CAKE

Prepare Chocolate Chiffon Cake but with the cocoa mixture sift:

| 1 tbsp. | (15 mL) | instant coffee |

Complete as for Chocolate Chiffon Cake.

STRAWBERRY SHORTCAKE

Prepare Plain Cake on page 83, but use a 7"x11" (18x28 cm) pan instead of an 8" (20 cm) square pan. Bake at 350°F (180°C), until a toothpick inserted in the centre comes out clean, 25-30 minutes. Turn pan upside down on wire rack until cool, about 45 minutes.

Wash and hull:
    1 qt. (1 L)   fresh strawberries

Reserve 10 perfect berries for garnishing. Slice remaining berries. Add to berries and mix well:
    5 tbsp. (75 mL)   unsweetened concentrated apple juice, defrosted

Beat until soft peaks form:
    1 cup (250 mL)   whipping cream, chilled

Add and beat until blended:
    1 tsp. (5 mL)   unsweetened concentrated apple juice, defrosted

Be careful not to overbeat cream.

Cut cake into 10 equal rectangles. Split each into half horizontally and place on a serving plate. Spread bottom layer of cake with ½ of the sliced berries and juice and ½ of the whipped cream. Cover with top part of cake. Spread with remainder of berries, juice and whipped cream. Garnish each piece of cake with a reserved berry, whole or sliced. Serves 10.

STRAWBERRY PUFF RING

Oil a 12" or 13" (30 or 33 cm) pizza pan or a large cookie sheet.

In a heavy saucepan, heat until boiling:
    1 cup (250 mL)   unsweetened apple juice OR water
    ½ cup (125 mL)   butter OR margarine OR 6 tbsp. (90 mL) vegetable oil

Add all at once:
    1 cup (250 mL)   all-purpose flour

With a wooden spoon, stir vigorously until mixture forms a ball around spoon. Remove from heat. (Do not overcook or dough will not puff.)

STRAWBERRY PUFF RING (continued)

Beat in thoroughly, 1 at a time:
    4 (4) **eggs, room temperature**

Beat until mixture is thick, shiny and does not adhere to spoon.

Preheat oven to 400°F (200°C).

Use a tablespoon or a pastry bag fitted with a large fluted tube to transfer dough onto the prepared pan. If a pastry bag is used, hold the tube close to the pan. As you squeeze the bag, move your hand in tiny circular motions until a walnut-sized portion of dough forms a rosette. Make 12 rosettes, placing them on pan to form a circle. Allow space for expansion.

Bake 15 minutes at 400°F (200°C); reduce to 325°F (160°C) for 25-30 minutes. Remove from oven; cut rosettes horizontally into 2 layers. Cool. Fill bottom layer with half of Strawberry Topping, recipe follows. Cover with top layer. Pipe rosettes with remaining topping to decorate each puff. When ready to serve, cut whole strawberries into halves; place on each rosette. Makes 12 puffs.

See photograph on page 80A.

STRAWBERRY TOPPING

Combine; warm over low heat until dissolved:
    1 tbsp. (15 mL) **unsweetened concentrated apple juice, defrosted**
    1 tbsp (15 mL) **water**
    1½ tsp. (7 mL) **gelatine**

Add; mix well; chill until thick but not set:
    ⅓ cup (75 mL) **evaporated milk, 2% m.f.**

Wash, hull and crush:
    1 cup (250 mL) **sliced strawberries**

Add berries to thickened milk mixture with:
    3 tbsp. (45 mL) **unsweetened concentrated apple juice, defrosted**

Beat until light and fluffy. Makes 1¾ cups (425 ml).

Cookies, Bars and Squares

LACY ALMOND COOKIES

On a baking sheet, toast, see instructions page 85:
    ¾ cup   (175 mL)   slivered almonds

Combine in a small saucepan:
    5 tbsp. (75 mL)   unsweetened concentrated apple juice, defrosted
    2 tsp.   (10 mL)   orange rind, finely chopped
    10   (10)   pitted dates, finely chopped

Cook and stir over medium-low heat until thick and smooth. Remove from heat.

Add:
    3 tbsp. (45 mL)   butter OR margarine
    ¼ tsp. (1 mL)   almond extract

Stir in:
    4 tbsp. (60 mL)   evaporated milk

Sift together:
    4 tbsp. (60 mL)   all-purpose flour
    ¼ tsp. (1 mL)   baking soda

Add flour mixture to milk mixture; mix until blended. Stir in the toasted almonds. Drop teaspoonfuls of batter onto an oiled cookie sheet. Flatten with back of spoon. Bake at 350°F (180°C) until brown, 10-12 minutes. Makes 20 cookies.

FLORENTINES

Make Lacy Almond Cookies, see recipe page 94. Set aside until cooled.

Melt over low heat:
    3 oz. (85 g) unsweetened plain carob bar

Add:
    1 tbsp. (15 mL) butter OR margarine

Mix well. Remove from heat. Cool to lukewarm. Invert cooled cookies. With a spatula, spread the lukewarm carob mixture to cover bottoms of cookies. Allow to dry. Store or serve, right side up. Makes 20 cookies.

CAROB CHIP COOKIES

Cook and stir until thick and smooth; cool:
    14 (14) pitted dates, finely chopped
    ⅔ cup (150 mL) unsweetened concentrated fruit juice, any flavour, defrosted

Sift together:
    1½ cups (375 mL) all-purpose flour
    ¾ tsp. (4 mL) baking soda

To flour add:
    ½ cup (125 mL) carob chips, unsweetened
    ¼ cup (60 mL) chopped walnuts

Cream until soft and creamy:
    5 tbsp. (75 mL) butter OR margarine

Beat in thoroughly:
    1 (1) egg
    1 tsp. (5 mL) vanilla

Add date mixture to creamed mixture and beat until blended:

Mix in dry ingredients. Roll into small balls or drop from a small spoon. Place on an oiled cookie sheet. Flatten with lightly floured bottom of a tumbler. Bake at 350°F (180°C) until golden, about 15 minutes. Makes 3 dozen 2" (5 cm) cookies.

DIGESTIVE COOKIES

Cook and stir over medium heat until thick and smooth; cool:

14	(	14)	pitted dates, finely chopped
6 tbsp.	(	90 mL)	unsweetened concentrated apple juice, defrosted
6 tbsp.	(	90 mL)	unsweetened concentrated orange juice, defrosted

Sift together:

⅓ cup	(	75 mL)	unbleached OR all-purpose flour
¾ tsp.	(	4 mL)	baking powder
¾ tsp.	(	4 mL)	baking soda

Add:

½ cup	(	125 mL)	whole-wheat flour
¼ cup	(	60 mL)	wheat germ
2 tbsp.	(	30 mL)	natural bran
½ cup	(	125 mL)	quick-cooking rolled oats

Cream until soft and creamy:

| ½ cup | (| 125 mL) | butter OR margarine |

Beat in:

| 1 | (| 1) | egg |
| 1 tsp. | (| 5 mL) | vanilla |

Add cooled date mixture to creamed mixture; beat until blended. Stir in dry ingredients. Drop batter from a small spoon onto a lightly oiled cookie sheet. Flatten with tines of a fork. Bake at 350°F (180°C) until brown, 16-20 minutes. Makes thirty-four 2½" (6 cm) cookies.

TO BAKE COOKIES

Use a pan with very low sides or place cookies on an inverted pan. The heat will circulate freely over the cookies.

COFFEE DATE BARS

BASE AND TOPPING

Warm over low heat until hot:
- 2½ tbsp.   (37 mL)   **unsweetened concentrated apple juice, defrosted**

Stir into juice; set aside until cool:
- 2 tsp.   (10 mL)   **instant coffee**

Sift together:
- 1¼ cup   (300 mL)   **all-purpose flour**
- 1 tsp.   (5 mL)   **baking powder**

Cut into flour mixture with pastry blender until crumbly:
- ½ cup   (125 mL)   **butter OR margarine**

Add:
- ½ cup   (125 mL)   **chopped nuts**

Sprinkle flour mixture with the coffee liquid; mix well. Press about ⅔ flour mixture into an oiled 8" (20 cm) square pan. Cover with Date Filling, recipe follows. Spread remaining flour mixture on top, patting down lightly. Bake at 350°F (180°C) until light brown, about 25 minutes. Cool. Cut into 1"x 2" (2.5x5 cm) bars. Makes 32 bars.

DATE FILLING

Combine in a saucepan:
- ½ cup   (125 mL)   **hot water**
- 3 tsp.   (15 mL)   **instant coffee**
- ½ cup   (125 mL)   **unsweetened concentrated apple juice, defrosted**
- 1 cup   (250 mL)   **pitted dates, finely sliced**

Bring to a boil; then simmer and stir until thick and smooth; cool.

TO FOLD EGG WHITES

Fold egg whites into batter with a rubber spatula or plastic scraper using an up, over and down movement. Stirring egg whites into batter will drive out the air and make the egg whites collapse.

FRUIT BARS

BASE

Sift into a mixing bowl:
- 1 cup   (250 mL)   all-purpose flour
- 1 tsp.   (5 mL)   baking powder

Cut in with pastry blender until crumbly:
- 5 tbsp. (75 mL)   butter OR margarine

Sprinkle with:
- 2 tbsp. (30 mL)   unsweetened concentrated fruit juice, any flavour, defrosted

Mix well with a fork. Press into a lightly oiled 8" (20 cm) square pan. Bake at 350°F (180°C) for 15 minutes. Spread Fruit Filling, recipe follows, over prebaked base. Sprinkle over filling, patting down lightly:
- ¼ cup   (60 mL)   unsweetened shredded coconut

Bake until coconut is nicely browned, 20-25 minutes. Cool. Cut into 1"x 2" (2.5x5 cm) bars. Makes 32 bars.

FRUIT FILLING

Combine in a saucepan:
- 10   (10)   apricots, finely chopped
- 14   (14)   dates, finely chopped
- ⅓ cup   (75 mL)   figs, finely chopped
- ⅓ cup   (75 mL)   raisins
- 6 tbsp. (90 mL)   unsweetened concentrated fruit juice, any flavour, defrosted
- ⅔ cup   (150 mL)   water

Cook and stir over medium-low heat until all liquid is absorbed. Cool.

APRICOT BARS

Prepare Fruit Bars, page 98, but spread Apricot Filling over prebaked base. Complete as for Fruit Bars.

APRICOT FILLING

Combine in a saucepan:
- 1⅔ cups (400 mL) finely chopped dried apricots
- ⅔ cup (150 mL) unsweetened concentrated apple juice, defrosted
- ⅓ cup (75 mL) water
- 2 tsp. (10 mL) lemon juice

Cook and stir over medium-low heat until liquid is absorbed. Cool.

BROWNIES

Oil and lightly flour an 8" (20 cm) square cake pan. Melt over low heat and mix well:
- 2 oz. (57 g) unsweetened chocolate
- 3 tbsp. (45 mL) butter OR margarine

Preheat oven to 350°F (180°C). Sift together:
- 1 cup (250 mL) sifted all-purpose flour
- 1 tsp. (5 mL) baking powder
- ½ tsp. (2 mL) baking soda
- 1 tbsp. (15 mL) instant skim milk powder (press through a sieve)

Mix in:
- ¾ cup (175 mL) chopped walnuts

Beat well:
- 2 (2) large eggs

Beat chocolate mixture into eggs. Add; beat on low until blended:
- ½ tsp. (2 mL) vanilla
- ⅞ cup (205 mL) unsweetened concentrated apple juice, room temperature

Fold the flour mixture into the chocolate mixture. Pour into prepared pan. Bake about 35 minutes. Cut into 2" (5 cm) squares when cooled. Makes 16 brownies.

RAISIN SQUARES

BASE AND TOPPING

Sift into a mixing bowl:
- 1 cup (250 mL) all-purpose flour
- 1 tsp. (5 mL) baking powder

Add:
- ¼ cup (60 mL) fine soda cracker crumbs

Cut in with pastry blender until crumbly:
- ½ cup (125 mL) butter OR margarine

Sprinkle with:
- 2 tbsp. (30 mL) unsweetened concentrated orange juice, defrosted

Mix well with a fork. Press ⅔ of flour mixture into a lightly oiled 8" (20 cm) square pan. Cover with Raisin Filling, recipe follows. Spread remaining mixture on top, patting down lightly. Bake at 350°F (180°C) until light brown, about 35 minutes. Cool. Cut into squares. Makes twenty-five 1½" (3.8 cm) squares.

RAISIN FILLING

Combine in a saucepan until smooth:
- 1 tbsp. (15 mL) cornstarch
- 6 tbsp. (90 mL) unsweetened concentrated orange juice, defrosted
- 3 tbsp. (45 mL) water

Cook and stir over medium-low heat until filling thickens. Add:
- 1½ cups (375 mL) raisins

Cook and stir 2 minutes. Cool.

FIG SQUARES

BASE AND TOPPING

Combine:
- 1 cup (250 mL) whole-wheat OR all-purpose flour
- 1 tsp. (5 mL) baking powder

Add:
- 1 cup (250 mL) quick-cooking rolled oats

Cut in with pastry blender until crumbly:
- 6 tbsp. (90 mL) butter OR margarine

Sprinkle:
- 2 tbsp. (30 mL) unsweetened concentrated orange juice, defrosted

Mix well. Press about ½ of this mixture into an oiled 8" square (20 cm) pan. Cover with Fig Filling, recipe follows. Spread remaining mixture on top, patting down lightly. Bake at 350°F (180°C) until nicely browned, about 35 minutes. Cool. Makes twenty-five 1½" (3.8 cm) squares.

FIG FILLING

Wash in hot water; drain;
- ½ lb. (250 g) figs

With scissors, snip off the stems, then snip figs into small pieces.

Combine in a small saucepan:
- 1 tbsp. (15 mL) all-purpose flour
- ½ cup (125 mL) unsweetened concentrated orange juice, defrosted
- ¾ cup (175 mL) water

Add the figs. Simmer and stir 10 minutes. Cool.

Treats

CHOCOLATE-DIPPED FRUITS

Melt over low heat:
    1 oz. (**30 g**) unsweetened chocolate

Add and mix until blended:
    5 tbsp. (**75 mL**) unsweetened concentrated apple juice, defrosted

Cook and stir chocolate mixture over medium-low heat until it thickens, 5-7 minutes.

Add:
    1 tsp. (**5 mL**) butter OR margarine

Remove from heat. Add:
    ½ tsp. (**2 mL**) vanilla

Cool to lukewarm.

Use any of the following fruits for dipping:
- **strawberries with stems attached**, wash and pat dry;
- **dried apricots, wash and pat dry;**
- **pineapple rings, cut into wedges** and pat dry;
- **sliced bananas, dip in lemon juice** and allow to dry.

Dip fruits individually into lukewarm chocolate to half-coat each fruit. Place on a wire rack; chill. Makes about 3 dozen Chocolate-Dipped Fruits.

CHOCOLATE NUT CLUSTERS

Bring to a boil, then simmer and stir until thick and smooth; cool;
- ⅓ cup (75 mL) unsweetened concentrated apple juice, defrosted
- 10 (10) dates, finely sliced

Sift together:
- 6 tbsp. (90 mL) all-purpose flour
- 2 tbsp. (30 mL) cocoa
- ¼ tsp. (1 mL) baking powder
- ¼ tsp. (1 mL) baking soda

Beat the cooled date mixture well with:
- 2 tbsp. (30 mL) butter OR margarine
- 1 (1) egg
- 1 tsp. (5 mL) vanilla

Fold the flour mixture into the date mixture and stir in:
- 2 cups (500 mL) nuts (walnuts, pecans, almonds OR mixed nuts)

Drop batter, about the size of a walnut, from a small spoon, onto a lightly oiled cookie sheet. Bake at 350°F (180°C) for 11 minutes. Makes 32 clusters.

CHOCOLATE COCONUT CLUSTERS

Prepare Chocolate Nut Clusters but instead of nuts fold in the flour mixture and:
- 1¾ cups (425 mL) unsweetened shredded coconut

Drop small mounds of coconut mixture from a small spoon onto a lightly oiled cookie sheet. Bake at 350°F (180°C) until brown, about 15-20 minutes. Makes 3 dozen Chocolate Coconut Clusters.

FLUFFY "MARSHMALLOWS"

Lightly dust a 7"x11" (18x28 cm) pan with cornstarch.

Soak in a small mixing bowl and set aside:
- 3 tbsp. (45 mL) gelatine (3 envelopes)
- ½ cup (125 mL) hot (not boiling) water

In a heavy saucepan over medium-high heat, cook, without stirring, until thermometer registers 240°F (120°C):
- 1¼ cups (300 mL) unsweetened concentrated pineapple juice, defrosted

Remove juice from heat; pour over soaked gelatine; stir until combined. Beat on high speed until thick, 15 minutes. Add and beat until blended:
- 1 tsp. (5 mL) vanilla

Pour into prepared pan. When set (about 4 hours), slice into squares by cutting 5 rows across and 8 rows down; dust lightly with:
- cornstarch

Store in a covered tin box. Makes 40 "marshmallows."

LEMON JELLIES

Combine in a cup:
- 5 tbsp. (75 mL) unsweetened concentrated apple juice, defrosted
- 6 tbsp. (90 mL) water
- 3 tbsp. (45 mL) gelatine (3 envelopes)

Heat to boiling point:
- 1½ cups (375 mL) unsweetened pineapple juice
- 4 tbsp. (60 mL) lemon juice
- 1 tsp. (5 mL) grated lemon rind

Stir gelatine mixture into pineapple juice mixture until gelatine has completely dissolved. Pour into an 8" (20 cm) square pan. Chill until firm. Slice into rectangular pieces by cutting 6 rows across and 10 rows down.*

Blend until very fine:
- 2 tbsp. (30 mL) unsweetened shredded coconut, toasted

LEMON JELLIES (continued)

Roll each jelly in the blended coconut. Refrigerate until ready to serve. Makes 60 slices.

* For special occasions, use cookie cutters to make hearts, stars, etc.

ORANGE JELLIES

Combine in a cup:
¾ cup (	175 mL)	**unsweetened orange juice**
3 tbsp. (	45 mL)	**gelatine (3 envelopes)**

Heat to boiling point:
1⅔ cup (	400 mL)	**unsweetened orange juice**
1 tsp. (	5 mL)	**grated orange rind**

Stir gelatine mixture into orange juice mixture until gelatine has completely dissolved. Continue as for Lemon Jellies.

GRAPE JELLIES

Instead of unsweetened orange juice and grated orange rind use:
unsweetened grape juice (red OR purple)

PINEAPPLE JELLIES

Instead of unsweetened orange juice and grated orange rind use:
unsweetened pineapple juice

BANANA YOGURT POPSICLES

Mix with a fork:
    1 (1) large banana, mashed
    1 tbsp. (15 mL) unsweetened concentrated apple juice, defrosted

Fold in:
    1½ cups (375 mL) yogurt

Spoon into 8 popsicle moulds or paper cups. Freeze until firm. If paper cups are used, insert popsicle sticks when partially frozen; then freeze until firm.

To remove popsicles from moulds, immerse in warm water until loosened. To remove individually, invert mould. Wrap a hot towel around 1 unit, until a popsicle slides out. Yields 8 popsicles.

VARIATIONS:

Replace banana with:
    ½ cup (125 mL) puréed peaches, pears, apples, pineapple (if canned, drain well), OR crushed berries.

ORANGE POPSICLES

Pour into 8 popsicle moulds or paper cups:
    2 cups (500 mL) unsweetened orange juice

Freeze until firm. If paper cups are used, insert popsicle sticks when partially frozen; then freeze until firm.

To remove popsicles from moulds, immerse in warm water until loosened. To remove individually, invert mould. Wrap hot towel around 1 unit, until a popsicle slides out. Yields 8 popsicles.

VARIATIONS:

Replace unsweetened orange juice with:
    2 cups (500 mL) unsweetened red OR purple grape juice, unsweetened pineapple juice, OR apple juice.

INDEX

Apple
  Apple-Cheddar Coffee Cake...............11
  Apple Coleslaw 25
  Apple-Cranberry Sauce 49
  Apple Horseradish Relish 55
  Apple Pie 66
  Apple Pork Chops 39
  Tangy Apple Wedges 38
Baked Beans 38
Black Forest Cake 80
Bread & Butter Pickles 53
Brownies 99

CAKES
  Apple-Cheddar Coffee Cake 11
  Black Forest Cake 80
  Chiffon Cakes
    Chocolate Chiffon Cake 91
    Lemon Chiffon Cake........................88
    Maple Walnut Chiffon Cake 90
    Mocha Chiffon Cake 91
    Orange Chiffon Cake.......................88
    Poppy Seed Chiffon Cake 89
    Vanilla Chiffon Cake 90
  Lemon-Raisin Bundt Cake 10
  Marble Cake 82
  Orange Cake 86
  Plain Cake 83
  Poppy Seed Torte 84
  Strawberry Puff Ring 92
  Strawberry Shortcake 92
Cheese
  Apple-Cheddar Coffee Cake...............11
  Cheese Puffs 19
  Lemon Cheesecake 79
  No-Bake Fruit Cheesecake 78
  Rolled Cheesewiches 16
Chocolate
  Brownies 99
  Chocolate Chiffon Cake 91
  Chocolate Coconut Clusters 103
  Chocolate Dessert Pancakes 9
  Chocolate-Dipped Fruits 102
  Chocolate Nut Clusters 103
  Chocolate Sauce 61

  Chocolate Whipped Cream 85
  Low-Calorie Chocolate Topping 9
Cooked Salad Dressing.........................23

COOKIES, BARS & SQUARES
  Bars
    Apricot Bars..................................99
    Coffee Date Bars 97
    Fruit Bars 98
  Cookies
    Carob Chip Cookies 95
    Digestive Cookies 96
    Florentines 95
    Lacy Almond Cookies.....................94
  Squares
    Brownies......................................99
    Fig Squares 101
    Raisin Squares 100
Cranberry
  Apple-Cranberry Sauce 49
  Cranberry Chutney............................51
  Cranberry Jelly 50
  Cranberry Sauce 50
  Spiced Cranberry Sauce 50
Crusts
  Pizza Crust 45
  Tender Pie Pastry..............................62
  Whole-Wheat Pizza Crust 34
Curried Lamb 37
Custard Cream for trifles 73
Custard Cream Filling for cakes............84

FILLINGS
  Apricot Filling 18, 99
  Cheese Filling for Cheesewiches........17
  Coffee Date Filling 97
  Custard Cream for Trifles 73
  Custard Cream Filling for Cakes.........84
  Fig Filling 101
  Fruit Filling 98
  Orange Filling & Topping for Cakes...87
  Poppy Seed Filling 14
  Raisin Filling 100
Florentines 95
French Dressing 21

FROSTINGS, TOPPINGS & GLAZES

Carob Curls 81
Glaze
   Pineapple Glaze 40
Meringue
   Lemon Meringue................................68
   Nut Meringue 69
   Pineapple Meringue 67
Orange Filling and Topping................87
Strawberry Topping 93
Whipped Cream
   Chocolate Whipped Cream 85
   Low-Calorie Chocolate Topping..........9
   Whipped Cream 73
Fruit Bars..98
Fruit Filling...98
Glazed Carrot..31
Grape Jellies.......................................105
Green Tomato Pickles.........................52
Ham, Pineapple Glazed......................39
Harvard Beets 31
Hawaiian Meatballs.............................35
Hot Cross Buns 15

JAMS

Peach Jam 58
Plum Jam 59
Rhubarb-Pineapple Jam 57
Rhubarb-Strawberry Jam 57
Strawberry Jam 58
Lacy Almond Cookies...........................94
Lemon
   Lemon-Raisin Bundt Cake 10
   Lemon Cheesecake 79
   Lemon Chicken 42
   Lemon Chiffon Cake 88
   Lemon Jellies 104
   Lemon Meringue 68
   Lemon Pie 68
   Lemon Pudding 75
   Lemon Snow 75
   Self-Saucing Lemon Pudding.............77
Low-Calorie Chocolate Topping............9
Low-Calorie Mayonnaise 22

MAIN DISHES

Baked Beans 38
Beef
   Beef Pizza 34
   Beef Tomato 32
   Cabbage Rolls.....................................36
   Hawaiian Meatballs 35
   Sauerbraten 33
Fish
   Sweet & Sour Fish 44
   Tuna Pizza 45
Lamb, Curried.......................................37
Pork
   Apple Pork Chops 39
   Barbecued Spareribs 40
   Ham, Pineapple Glazed.....................39
   Sweet and Sour Spareribs 41
Poultry
   Lemon Chicken 42
   Orange Barbecued Chicken..............43
   Pineapple Chicken 42
   Roast Duck À L'Orange 44
Maple Walnut Chiffon Cake................90
Maple Sauce 61
"Marshmallows", Fluffy 104
Meringue
   Lemon Meringue 68
   Nut Meringue 69
   Pineapple Meringue 67
Mexican Crêpes 8
Mocha Chiffon Cake 91

MUFFINS

Banana Nut Bran Muffins......................6
Oatmeal Muffins 6
Pumpkin Muffins 5
Rice-Bacon Muffins 7
Rice-Raisin Muffins 7
Mustard Bean Pickle 52
No-Bake Fruit Cheesecake 79
Orange
   Orange Barbecue Sauce for Chicken ..43
   Orange Barbecued Chicken 43
   Orange Cake 86
   Orange Chiffon Cake 88
   Orange Filling & Topping 87
   Orange Jellies 105

Orange Popsicles 106
Orange Sauce...................................60
Roast Duck À L'Orange......................44
Self-Saucing Orange Pudding............77

PANCAKES, CRÊPES

Chocolate Dessert Pancakes 9
Mexican Crêpes 8
Rice Pancakes....................................8

PASTRY, PIES & CRUSTS

Crusts & Pastry
  Pizza Crust...................................45
  Tender Pie Pastry 62
  Whole-Wheat Pizza Crust................34
Pies
  Apple Pie 66
  Blueberry Pie................................66
  Lemon Pie 68
  Peach Pie 63
  Pumpkin Chiffon Pie 70
  Raisin Meringue Pie 69
  Rhubarb Bavarian Pie 64
  Rhubarb-Strawberry Pie 65
  Sour Cream Pineapple Pie..............67
  Strawberry Bavarian Pie 64
Peach
  Peach Chutney..............................51
  Peach Jam 58
  Peach Pie 63
  Peach Sauce 59
Pear Sauce 60

PICKLES & RELISHES & SAUCES

Chili Sauce using canned tomatoes ...49
Chili Sauce using fresh tomatoes.......48
Chutney, Cranberry............................51
Chutney, Peach 51
Ketchup I, Tomato 46
Ketchup II, Tomato 47
Pickles
  Bread & Butter Pickles 53
  Green Tomato Pickles....................52
  Mustard Bean Pickles 52
  Pickled Beets 55
  Pickled Onions 54
Relishes
  Apple-Horseradish Relish................55
  Quick Beet Relish..........................54

Zucchini Relish..................................56

PIZZA

Beef Pizza..34
Pizza Crust 45
Tuna Pizza 45
Whole-Wheat Pizza Crust 34

Plain Cake 83
Plum Jam 59

PUDDINGS & CHEESECAKES

Cheesecakes
  Lemon Cheesecake........................79
  No-Bake Fruit Cheesecake 78
Puddings
  Carrot Pudding 76
  Creamy Rice Pudding.....................74
  Lemon Pudding.............................75
  Lemon Snow.................................75
  Pineapple Trifle 72
  Pumpkin Pudding..........................76
  Self-Saucing Lemon Pudding.........77
  Self-Saucing Orange Pudding 77
  Steamed Rhubarb..........................74
  Strawberry Trifle 71

Quick Beet Relish.............................54
Rhubarb
  Rhubarb-Pineapple Jam 57
  Rhubarb-Strawberry Jam 57
  Rhubarb Bavarian Pie 64
  Rhubarb-Strawberry Pie 65
  Steamed Rhubarb 74

Roast Duck À L'Orange......................44
Rolled Cheesewiches.........................16

SALAD AND FRUIT DRESSINGS

Cooked Salad Dressing 23
Cottage Cheese Fruit Dressing 24
Cottage Cheese Horseradish
Dressing 23
French Dressing................................21
Low-Calorie Mayonnaise....................22
Sour Cream Dressing 21
Sour Cream Horseradish Dressing......22
Thousand Island Dressing 22
Whipped Cream Fruit Salad
Dressing 24

109

SAUCES

Savoury Sauces
Apple-Cranberry Sauce.....................49
Barbecue Sauce for Spareribs..........40
Chili Sauce I..................................48
Chili Sauce II.................................49
Cranberry Jelly...............................50
Cranberry Sauce 50
Orange Barbecue Sauce for Chicken.43
Spiced Cranberry Sauce 50
Sweet & Sour Pineapple Sauce........41
Sweet & Sour Sauce 41
Tomato Ketchup I...........................46
Tomato Ketchup II..........................47

Sweet Sauces
Chocolate Sauce..............................61
Maple Sauce...................................61
Orange Sauce 60
Peach Sauce...................................59
Pear Sauce.....................................60

Sauerbraten 33
Self-Saucing Lemon Pudding 77
Self-Saucing Orange Pudding 77
Spiced Cranberry Sauce 50
Spicy Red Cabbage 27
Steamed Rhubarb................................74

Strawberry
Rhubarb-Strawberry Jam 57
Rhubarb-Strawberry Pie 65
Strawberry Bavarian Pie...................64
Strawberry Jam 58
Strawberry Puff Ring 92
Strawberry Shortcake 92
Strawberry Topping 93
Strawberry Trifle 71

Tangy Apple Wedges...........................38
Tender Pie Pastry 62
Thousand Island Dressing 22
Toasted Almonds.................................85

Tomato
Beef Tomato....................................32
Chili Sauce I....................................48
Chili Sauce II...................................49
Green Tomato Pickles 52
Tomato Ketchup I.............................46
Tomato Ketchup II............................47

TREATS
Banana Yogurt Popsicles..................106
Chocolate Coconut Clusters 103
Chocolate-Dipped Fruits 102
Chocolate Nut Clusters 103
Fluffy "Marshmallows" 104
Grape Jellies 105
Lemon Jellies 104
Orange Jellies 105
Orange Popsicles 106
Pineapple Jellies 105

Tuna Pizza 45
Vanilla Chiffon Cake............................90

VEGETABLES
Beans, Baked 38
Beans, Sweet & Sour 29
Beets, Harvard................................31
Carrots, Glazed...............................31
Coleslaw..25
Coleslaw Apple...............................25
Potato Salad 26
Red Cabbage, Spicy 27
Red Cabbage, Sweet & Sour............28
Squash, Glazed...............................30
Turnips, Baked 29
Turnips, Mashed 30
Whole-Wheat Pizza Crust.................34

YEAST BREADS, BUNS & CAKES
Apple-Cheddar Coffee Cake..............11
Apricot Log 17
Cheese Puffs..................................19
Hot Cross Buns...............................15
Lemon-Raisin Bundt Cake 10
Pizza Crust 45
Poppy Seed Ring 13
Rolled Cheesewiches 16
Seed & Grain Bread 20
Zucchini Relish................................56

SHARE **THE SUGARLESS COOKBOOKS** WITH A FRIEND

THE SUGARLESS COOKBOOKS are **$11.95** per book, plus $2.50 (total order) for shipping and handling:

The Sugarless Cookbook, Volume 1 _____	x $11.95	$_____
The Sugarless Cookbook, Volume 2 _____	x $11.95	$_____
Add shipping and handling charge_____		$ 2.50
Subtotal_____		$_____
In Canada add 7% Goods & Services Tax (GST) ___(Subtotal x .07)		$_____
Total enclosed_____		$_____

NAME: _____

STREET: _____

CITY: _____ **PROV./STATE** _____

COUNTRY _____ **POSTAL CODE/ZIP** _____

Please make cheque or money order payable to: **HUM Publishing**
                                                395 Second Avenue
                                                Ottawa, Ontario
                                                Canada K1S 2J3
                                                Telephone (613) 232-7295

Price subject to change / U.S. and International orders payable in U.S. funds

For fund raising or volume purchases, contact HUM Publishing for volume rates

---

SHARE **THE SUGARLESS COOKBOOKS** WITH A FRIEND

THE SUGARLESS COOKBOOKS are **$11.95** per book, plus $2.50 (total order) for shipping and handling:

The Sugarless Cookbook, Volume 1 _____	x $11.95	$_____
The Sugarless Cookbook, Volume 2 _____	x $11.95	$_____
Add shipping and handling charge_____		$ 2.50
Subtotal_____		$_____
In Canada add 7% Goods & Services Tax (GST) ___(Subtotal x .07)		$_____
Total enclosed_____		$_____

NAME: _____

STREET: _____

CITY: _____ **PROV./STATE** _____

COUNTRY _____ **POSTAL CODE/ZIP** _____

Please make cheque or money order payable to: **HUM Publishing**
                                                395 Second Avenue
                                                Ottawa, Ontario
                                                Canada K1S 2J3
                                                Telephone (613) 232-7295

Price subject to change/U.S. and International orders payable in U.S. funds

For fund raising or volume purchases, contact HUM Publishing for volume rates